DOCTORS OF CONSCIENCE

CAROLE JOFFE

Doctors of Conscience

THE STRUGGLE TO PROVIDE ABORTION
BEFORE AND AFTER *ROE V. WADE*

Beacon Press
Boston

Beacon Press
25 Beacon Street
Boston, Massachusetts 02108-2892

Beacon Press books
are published under the auspices of
the Unitarian Universalist Association of Congregations.

Portions of chapters 1, 2, and 4 originally appeared, in slightly different form, as
"Portraits of Three 'Physicians of Conscience': Abortion before Legalization in the
United States," *Journal of the History of Sexuality* 2 (1991): 46–67, and "The Unending
Struggle for Legal Abortion: Conversations with Jane Hodgson," *Journal of the
American Medical Women's Association* 49 (1994): 160–64.

99 98 97 96   8 7 6 5 4 3 2

Text design by Wesley B. Tanner/Passim Editions
Composition by Wilsted & Taylor

LIBRARY OF CONGRESS CATALOGING-IN-PUBLICATION DATA

Joffe, Carole E.
    Doctors of conscience : the struggle to provide abortion before and after
Roe v. Wade / Carole Joffe.
        p.   cm.
    Includes bibliographical references and index.
    ISBN 0-8070-2100-8 (cloth)
    ISBN 0-8070-2101-6 (paper)
    1. Abortion – Moral and ethical aspects.   2. Abortion – Social aspects – United
States.   3. Physicians – United States – Attitudes.
    I. Title.
HQ767.15.J64   1995
363.4'6 – dc20   95-11851
                                                                        CIP

Contents

Preface   vii

Acknowledgments   xv

Introduction   1

1   "I've Been Lucky to Have Been Part of This":   8
     Jane Hodgson and the Unending Struggle for Legal Abortion

2   U.S. Medicine and the Marginalization of Abortion   27

3   "The Lengths to Which Women Would Go":   53
     Encountering Abortion before *Roe*

4   "I Was Doing It for Reasons of Conscience":   70
     Providing Illegal Abortions

5   "I Wanted to Do Something about Abortion":   108
     Facilitating Abortions before *Roe*

6   "Getting Your Hands Dirty":   143
     The Practice of Legal Abortion

7   Assuring a Future for Legal Abortion   183

     Afterword   209

     Notes   211

     Index   243

Preface

The "back alley butcher" is the dominant image that has been used – by both supporters and opponents of abortion – to describe abortion providers in the pre-*Roe* era. The term is often used synonymously with "criminal abortionist." These phrases, used to refer both to medical and lay providers, evoke greedy, incompetent, and exploitative individuals, who often injured their patients, sometimes sexually abused them, and occasionally, due to their ineptness, even killed them. Along with its other dominant symbol of the "bad old days" – the coat hanger, which represents the lengths women would go to in attempts at self-abortion – the pro-choice movement has used the figure of the "butcher" as a warning of women's vulnerability when abortion is illegal. Neither the coat hanger nor the butcher are invented symbols. Women did in fact try to abort using hangers (among many other similarly dangerous objects), and we have ample accounts of women's harrowing encounters with butchers, both lay and physician. Indeed this book at numerous points adds to the documentation of both the incompetence and the dubious ethics of those who offered illegal abortions before *Roe*.

But such butchers/criminal abortionists were only one aspect of a more complex reality that formed the culture of illegal abortion. Abortion before *Roe* also drew the attention of another category of physicians, those I refer to as "physicians of conscience." In contrast to the butchers who had medical degrees, these physicians of conscience were not incompetent medically (and hence unable to function in mainstream medicine), did not appear to have performed

VII

abortions primarily for financial reasons, and were not exploitative of their patients. Like all physicians who offered abortions in that era, this group risked both imprisonment and loss of medical license, but given that these providers were already well-established in mainstream medical careers, they arguably risked more by their actions. The motivation for becoming involved in abortion on the part of this group was their compassion for the women with unwanted pregnancies facing an untenable situation – including their vulnerability to treatment by butchers.

I decided to write this book because of my scholarly interest in the societal regulation of reproductive behavior, as well as my personal belief that legal and accessible abortion is a necessary component of women's health care. As a student of the abortion issue, I noted that while there is a considerable amount of scholarship on those factors that led to the criminalization of abortion in the United States in the late nineteenth century, relatively little has been written on the actual circumstances of the many illegal abortions that took place before the *Roe v. Wade* decision legalized the procedure in 1973. As a supporter of the abortion rights movement, I was concerned that popular discourse about this pre-*Roe* activity – including the imagery utilized by the movement itself – was in certain ways inadequate, even distorted, in ways that were actually harmful to the pro-choice cause.

It is beyond dispute that many abortions took place in the United States while the procedure was illegal; some estimates put the number of abortions in the years leading up to *Roe* as high as 1.2 million. Many, probably a majority of these cases, were women's attempts at self-abortion. The others were performed by some combination of lay persons, nurses, midwives, and physicians.[1] How subsequent generations have come to *reconstruct* this culture of illegal abortion, and particularly to interpret the motivations and capabilities of those who performed abortions, is more problematical.

I began this study, therefore, in the late 1980s by locating and interviewing physicians who had performed illegal abortions before *Roe* for reasons of conscience. In simplest terms, my original purpose was to document a largely untold aspect of the pre-*Roe* era and, as suggested, to demonstrate that not all those who provided abor-

tions in that period deserved to be categorized as butchers. But as is
fortunately often the case in studies that depend on in-depth qualitative interviewing, my initial respondents led me to reconceive this
study in two ways. First, it quickly became clear that the story of abortion provision before *Roe* was far more rich and complex than the
simple question of whether a particular doctor had "done" abortions
or not. I became aware of a continuum of activities related to abortion
that those I considered conscience physicians undertook. Those who
stopped short of performing illegal abortions nevertheless took part
in a range of activities – some of which were also illegal – to help
women obtain abortions. These activities included locating reliable
providers of illegal abortions for their patients, providing consultations and medications to lay abortionists, providing back-up medical
services to recipients of illegal abortions, and working within the
medical community and the larger society for the legalization of
abortion. A number of those I ultimately interviewed played especially influential roles in developing protocols for abortion services
as various individual states began to legalize in the period immediately before *Roe*. Some of those I interviewed, once I expanded my
definition of the interview pool, had performed abortions which
were difficult to classify as either "legal" or "illegal" – the so-called
gray area abortions of the pre-*Roe* era, approved by hospital committees, but theoretically subject to review by legal authorities.

The subjects of this study also quickly led me to understand that I
had overstated the significance of the divide represented by the *Roe*
decision of 1973. While my initial interest had been exclusively in the
period before *Roe*, those I interviewed appeared as eager to discuss
their professional experiences *after* the legalization of abortion as
before it. In listening to their narratives, I began to realize how much
the history of illegal provision in the pre-*Roe* era – especially the negative image of the "abortionist" – continued to inform the practice of
legal abortion after *Roe*. I was most of all struck by the bittersweet
quality of many of the interviews. These physicians, all of whom had
undergone certain risks by their abortion activity before *Roe*, had
every reason to assume that the "abortion problem" would be solved
by legalization. And of course, in certain fundamental respects, it
was. Women no longer died or sustained serious injuries from illegal

abortions; physicians like themselves no longer had to fear arrest for performing or facilitating abortions. Yet, in ways utterly unanticipated by this group, their continued commitment to providing abortion after legalization came at a considerable price. This price has included not only harassment by the antiabortion movement – which was just entering a particularly violent phase at the time of these interviews – but also, for many, isolation and stigmatization within the medical community. Thus, the scope of this study came to include providers' experiences after legalization as well.

This book draws on interviews I conducted with forty-five individuals whom I consider "physicians of conscience." Initially, I located respondents for this study in various ways, including making inquiries at professional associations and placing advertisements in medical journals. As the study progressed, one of my key ways of locating respondents was the "snowball" technique – that is, those whom I interviewed would recommend colleagues who they felt would be appropriate for this research.

The interview pool consists of thirty-five men and ten women. At the time of the interviews, the age of the respondents ranged from eighty to forty-eight, with the majority in their fifties and sixties. Three of the men interviewed are African-American. Thirty-six of those interviewed are obstetrician-gynecologists (ob/gyns), and the remainder are family practitioners. While fifteen of this group performed illegal abortions before *Roe*, and the rest engaged in various supplementary activities, all of them provided abortions after *Roe*. Eight of those interviewed had already retired from medical practice, while a larger group described themselves as "near retirement." While Jane Hodgson, the subject of chapter 1, and Henry Morgentaler, whose case is described in chapter 4, are identified because of the public nature of their arrests and subsequent trials, I have used fictional names for all of the others interviewed and have changed various identifying details, including geographical locations.*

*With respect to other names that appear in the text, I have usually changed the names of those mentioned by interviewees, unless the activity under discussion was a matter of public record. I have indicated those instances in which I have used fictional names other than those of the interviewees.

The dividing-line between "physicians of conscience" and the "butcher/criminal abortionist" of the pre-*Roe* era is not always clear, of course. In seeking physicians to interview for this book, I looked for those who lacked the characteristics most strongly associated with the butcher, who was greedy, incompetent, and unethical. But making these judgments – on the basis of informants' recollections of activities that took place from twenty to fifty years ago – was hardly a straightforward matter. "Greed" was perhaps the easiest issue to deal with. Of the subset of fifteen I interviewed who had performed illegal abortions, I asked about fees. Most had charged for this service, while several had not. Of those who accepted fees, all did so at rates considerably less than what the most high-priced abortionists of the period charged ($1000 or more), and all of them moreover had sliding scales and offered abortions free to indigent women. Indeed, some among this group told me that one of their motivations in providing abortions was to protect women from the "outrageous" fees demanded by others.

Incompetence and dubious ethics are far more difficult to assess when depending solely on the self-reports of individuals. Some who performed illegal abortions acknowledged some difficulties when they first began, difficulties which are understandable in light of the absence of training in abortion technique and the lack of colleagues with whom to discuss this work. None reported losing a patient or seriously injuring her. The various breaches of ethics reported from the pre-*Roe* period – ranging from operating under the influence of drugs or alcohol and demanding sexual favors from the patient to working in unsanitary and unsafe conditions – are not reflected in the narratives offered by those I interviewed (though one would hardly expect someone to volunteer such information).

Therefore, in selecting interview subjects, I decided to seek physicians active in the pre-*Roe* era who were already launched in seemingly successful mainstream medical careers. Such individuals, it was reasonable to assume, were not involved in abortion primarily for financial reasons, nor because they simply couldn't function successfully in other "above ground" aspects of medicine. On the contrary, it was mainstream physicians such as these who arguably had the most to lose and hence I assumed that their involvement was motivated by "conscience."

To be sure, the contrast of the "good" physician with the "bad" butcher/criminal abortionist is a highly simplified (and ultimately incomplete) account of abortion provision before *Roe*. As Rickie Solinger has compellingly argued in her recent work, many lay women abortionists active in that period were highly competent (based on known death and injury rates), and seemingly ethical as well.[2] Furthermore, many of the pre-*Roe* physicians who were involved in full-time abortion provision (and thus for whom this work represented a "living" as opposed to a conscience-driven "calling") were similarly medically and ethically sound; but it is the butchers – who in numerical terms were a minority of all providers – who have come to represent in the popular imagination all those who performed abortions before *Roe*. I am not suggesting, therefore, that the physicians of conscience, the subjects of this book, represent the only true "heroes" (from a pro-choice perspective) of the pre-*Roe* era. Rather, I argue that because of their strong links to mainstream medicine, the experiences of this group are particularly useful for understanding the development of abortion services in the United States. It was this group, more than other categories of pre-*Roe* abortion providers, that pushed for legalization both within medical circles and larger political arenas. It was from within "conscience" circles that the first generation of pro-choice medical leaders was drawn – those who pressured their hospitals to establish abortion services, helped to found the first freestanding clinics, wrote the textbooks on abortion techniques, and so forth. And it is the experiences of these doctors, whose careers so often reflect the price they paid for their commitment to abortion provision, that tells us the most about the difficult history and uncertain place that abortion services have had within the larger medical establishment.

The time period of these interviews deserves additional mention. Most of the interviews took place during the late 1980s (while a few occurred during the early 1990s). While antiabortion harassment of providers and patients started to increase considerably during the late 1980s, it would not be till a few years later that the worst manifestations of this campaign of terror occurred – the firebombings, death threats, stalking incidents, shootings, and, ultimately, murders. In retrospect, I believe that because the majority of interviews preceded the worst of the antiabortion violence, both the interview subjects and I could more easily consider additional aspects of the predicament of abortion providers after *Roe*, such as the marginal status of abortion within most medical institutions.

In spite of the occasionally difficult, even painful, material that was raised in the course of the interviews, the physicians with whom I spoke appeared to find the interviews engaging. Several volunteered that they had not spoken of their pre-*Roe* activity for many years, if ever, and said that they had enjoyed the occasion – rare in busy practitioners' lives – to reflect on their work, both past and present. My own response to these interviews, at the time that they were done, was largely an intellectual one. I was fascinated both by the details of abortion provision in the pre-*Roe* era, as well as the accounts of their unanticipated struggles to legitimate abortion services after *Roe*. Not unexpectedly, I felt admiration for the integrity and courage of those whose stories I heard, but it was not until several years later that the full emotional significance of these interviews hit me. As antiabortion violence escalated in the early 1990s, it felt almost surreal to me that the thoughtful, compassionate health care professionals with whom I had earlier spoken were now being stalked and terrorized, and their workplaces destroyed. Like many other Americans – on both sides of the abortion issue – I am saddened and enraged at the level of terrorism that has now become commonplace for abortion-providing physicians, clinic staff, escorts, and abortion patients. With awe and gratitude, I salute those on the front lines of abortion provision who continue – in circumstances most of us would find unendurable – to work for women's health.

A NOTE ON TERMINOLOGY

As this preface has suggested, the term "abortionist" has been highly controversial, carrying strong connotations of greed, ineptness, and unethical practices. Many use "abortionist" and "butcher" synonymously in referring to the pre-*Roe* era. Indeed, as several of the subjects of this book acknowledged, they themselves had to struggle to overcome negative images of the "abortionist." One of those interviewed, a third-generation ob/gyn, remarked, "In my family, the worst thing that could be said about anybody was that he was an abortionist." Given that one of the prime objectives of this book is precisely to show that not all those who provided abortions in the pre-*Roe* era merit such scorn, arguably this book should use "abortionist" in an affirmative manner, and attempt to restore dignity, or at least neutrality, to the term. While conceding a certain logic to that view, I have nonetheless come to agree with the position articulated by Warren Hern, M.D., who argues that the term is beyond reclamation. In a letter to the *New York Times*, complaining about the use of the word "abortionist" in a headline, Hern wrote, "There are some words that are so laden with historically stigmatized meanings that they cannot be separated from that context, no matter how hard people may try to bring them into accepted use."[5] Hence, throughout this book, in referring to those I interviewed, I will use the term "abortion provider" rather than "abortionist."

Acknowledgments

My greatest debt is to those physicians who agreed to my requests for interviews. To Jane Hodgson, Henry Morgentaler, and the others who appear in this book under pseudonyms, my heartfelt thanks for all you have taught me–about your work, and much more besides.

I am also very grateful to Terry Beresford, who has been my valued informant about the world of reproductive health services for nearly twenty years. Many of the ideas in this book were first developed in discussions with her, and she has generously permitted me to make use of several interviews she conducted with abortion providers. Throughout the course of this project, she has made herself available to read drafts, offer advice, and share with me her prodigious knowledge of abortion services in the United States.

This research was made possible by financial support I received from the Louis Stott Foundation and several faculty research grants from Bryn Mawr College and the University of California at Davis. A fellowship at the Davis Humanities Research Institute provided invaluable time for writing. For the special interest they took in this project, I am particularly thankful to Martha Stott Diener and to Judith Shapiro, former Provost of Bryn Mawr. Special thanks also to Nona Smith, grants administrator at Bryn Mawr, for her many acts of competence and kindness.

Rosalind Petchesky, Debbie Rogow, Rickie Solinger, and Judy Stacey–four friends whose own writing and activism in the realms of reproductive and sexual politics have long inspired me–all gave generously of their time to read a draft of this book. I have not taken all of their suggestions, but each of them has helped to make this a much stronger work than it would have been otherwise. I am very grateful also to Jean Hunt for all she has taught me over the years about reproductive politics and, especially, the situation of the abortion provider. Fred Block has spent countless hours reading drafts, discussing abortion services, and helping in every other way imaginable to bring this book to fruition.

Others who have patiently answered my many questions, read portions of the manuscript, sent me information, and in various other ways helped me include Stanley Henshaw, Patricia Anderson, Alice Abarbanel, Gina Shaw, David Grimes, Allan Rosenfeld, Philip Stubblefield, Kitty Kolbert, Mary Murrell, Ben Orlove, Jeff Escoffier, Ann Swidler, the late Hal Benenson, Renée Fox, Jane Caplan, Steven Sondheimer, Paul Joffe, and Frankie Weiser. I also thank the members of my reading group at Davis–Cynthia Brantley, Stephanie Shields, Lynn Roller, Suad Joseph, Alison Berry, Francesca Miller, Anna Kuhn, Kari Lokke, and Vicki Smith–for their advice and encouragement.

Rachel Rubin, Eve Herschkopf, Ralene Walker, Eva Skuratowicz, and, especially, Anne Nurse served as effective and dedicated research assistants. Patricia Miller, Linda Bentley, and Brenda White did a similarly fine job in transcribing interview tapes. A special thank-you to Emanuel Fleiglman for lending me some very useful items from his library–for far longer than he (or I) thought I would need them. Thanks also to the librarians at the Schlesinger Library at Radcliffe College and the Sophia Smith Collection at Smith College.

At Beacon Press, Marya Van't Hul has been all an author could wish an editor to be, and I am very grateful for her sensitive and intelligent response to this book. I also thank Susan Meigs for her excellent job of copyediting.

Finally, I feel tremendous gratitude for the constant support I received during the writing of this book from my parents, siblings, and, especially, my husband and children. This book is dedicated to them with my love.

Introduction

In the early 1990s, many abortion rights supporters in the United States had come to fear that *Roe v. Wade*, the landmark Supreme Court decision legalizing abortion, would be overturned by an increasingly conservative Supreme Court. But to many onlookers' surprise, the Court's *Planned Parenthood v. Casey* decision in 1992, while upholding significant restrictions on abortion services, reaffirmed the essential finding of *Roe* that a woman has a constitutionally protected right to an abortion before the fetus is viable.[1] Later that year, Bill Clinton, who ran on a strong "pro-choice" platform, was elected president, and within his first two years in office, he had the opportunity to appoint two new justices, each with a record of support for *Roe*, to the Supreme Court. The *Casey* decision and Clinton's subsequent Court appointments mean that abortion – *albeit* in highly restricted form – will presumably remain legal for the foreseeable future. But from a pro-choice perspective, this legal victory may prove to be a hollow one. Abortion may remain legal, but for an increasing number of American women, it may well become inaccessible.

This gap between the legal status of abortion and the disturbing realities of contemporary abortion provision was very evident to me when I attended the annual meeting of the National Abortion Federation, an organization of abortion providers, in the spring of 1992, shortly before the *Casey* decision was announced. Having grown up as the daughter of a cardiologist, I had some sense of what medical meetings were like. I can remember my father returning home from regional and national conferences, excited about the advances in his field, stimulated by meeting colleagues with differing approaches to problems in treating heart disease. As a college student, I had occasionally met him at such events, when they took place near my campus. But the NAF meeting had a different character than other medical conferences I was familiar with. To be sure, there was the same lively exchange about appropriate techniques and protocols, the same "state of the art" presentations from recognized leaders in the field that presumably characterize all good medical meetings. But hovering over each session of the NAF meetings was a sense of the extraordinary embattled and precarious status of abortion provision.

One can argue of course that given the uncertainties of health reform and the rising concerns about malpractice, *any* medical conference in the 1990s would appear more beleaguered than the calmer events my father's generation of physicians attended in the 1950s and 1960s. But even allowing for the current turbulence in medicine, the NAF meetings had features that made clear abortion's unique status within contemporary medical practice. At no other medical meetings, for example, does one hear, in casual hallway conversation among participants, one physician ask another if she is "wearing her b.p.v. [bulletproof vest] these days?" Similarly, other medical groups presumably do not have to devote time at their professional meetings to sessions in which lawyers give updates on various restrictions in effect against disruptions at medical workplaces and at physicians' homes, and agents of the Bureau of Alcohol, Tobacco and Firearms offer tips on how to protect facilities against firebombings.

Such efforts to protect themselves and their patients against attacks from antiabortion terrorists are only the most dramatic manifestations of the much broader struggle abortion providers face. At a mundane level, abortion providers are daily confronted with landlords who, fearing physical damage or other reprisals, refuse to extend leases on clinic and office facilities; medical supply firms who balk at doing business with those identified with abortion work; hospitals that yield to antiabortion pressure and close their abortion services. Physicians who provide abortions maintain a constant wariness about the possible retaliatory actions of their antiabortion colleagues. At the NAF meeting, at a session on the management of complications of first trimester abortions performed in freestanding clinics, one speaker cautioned that if a patient were sent to a local hospital under certain circumstances, "an antiabortion doctor might do a punitive hysterectomy." At the same session, another participant warned that if a particularly risky procedure was undertaken in emergency circumstances, and failed, it would not only harm the patient but the "movement" as well.

But the struggle facing this branch of medicine is most evident in the enormous difficulty many facilities have in finding an adequate supply of abortion providers. At the NAF meeting, some clinic administrators told of being able to offer abortion services only every other week. Other administrators recounted how they are forced to fly in physicians from halfway across the country in order to hold regular clinics. The director of one clinic related to colleagues that she recently sent out letters of inquiry to every single graduating resident of obstetrics and gynecology (ob/gyn) programs across the country and received no replies.

Such concerns expressed at the NAF meeting are reflective of a national crisis in abortion provision. Some 84 percent of all U.S. counties are without abortion facilities. The number of U.S. hospitals where abortions are performed decreased by 18 percent between 1988 and 1992, and less than one third of the nation's hospitals with the capability to perform abortions (defined as hospitals that offer obstetrical services) do so.[2] The majority of ob/gyns presently in practice do not perform abortions, and most residents in this specialty are not routinely being trained in abortion procedures. A national survey done in 1991 of ob/gyn residency programs found a longstanding trend of decreasing training in abortion to be continuing. The study revealed that only 12 percent of all such residencies routinely require training in first trimester abortion techniques and only 6 percent for second trimester abortions. (These programs allow opt-out clauses for those morally opposed to abortion.) About 50 percent of ob/gyn residencies offer first trimester abortion training on an elective basis, and the remaining 38 percent have no provisions for this training. A similar study, done recently at Columbia University, found that nearly half of all graduating residents in ob/gyn had completed their studies without ever having performed a first trimester abortion. This shortage of abortion providers is believed to be one significant factor contributing to the much commented on decline in the number of abortions performed annually in the United States that began in the early 1990s.[3]

How can we explain this situation – that abortion is legal but increasingly inaccessible for many American women? The public health benefits of legal abortion have been amply documented. In contrast to the pre-*Roe* era, in which many thousands of women died or were injured from illegal abortions, legal abortion is among the safest procedures today performed in medicine; a recent report from the Council on Scientific Affairs of the American Medical Association quoted a rate of 0.4 deaths per 100,000 procedures.[4] And, despite the visibility of the antiabortion movement, polls have consistently shown a majority of the American people supporting legal abortion. While abortion polls are difficult to summarize, as respondents typically approve of abortion more under certain circumstances than others, one recent poll found that only 13 percent of those answering disapproved of abortions "under all circumstances." Another group of polls, taken in the months leading up to the *Webster v. Reproductive Health Services* case, the 1989 Supreme Court case that challenged *Roe*, found a solid majority of respondents opposed to overturning *Roe*. A similar level of support is true of U.S. physicians, including ob/gyns. In 1971, shortly before *Roe*, a poll of the membership of the American College of Obstetricians and Gynecologists revealed that 83 percent of those responding agreed that "elective abortions should be performed under some circumstances," and only 13 percent disagreed. When this poll was repeated in 1985, the numbers were virtually unchanged.[5]

In seeking to explain this puzzle – a high degree of support for legal abortion by both the general public and the medical specialty most directly affected, yet so little commitment by this specialty to provide necessary services and training – it is tempting to point to the violent wing of the antiabortion movement. As the above discussion of the NAF convention suggested, providers in the early 1990s were deeply preoccupied with the safety of their patients and themselves.

In 1988, 85 percent of the freestanding abortion clinics serving four hundred or more patients reported some form of antiabortion harassment. In 1992, there were almost two hundred recorded "violent" incidents at abortion facilities (a category including clinic or office invasions, acts of vandalism, arson, and bombings) and nearly three thousand incidents of "disruption" (hate mail and harassing calls, bomb threats, and picketing). One year later, in March 1993, the worst fears of abortion providers materialized when one of their colleagues, David Gunn, was killed in front of an abortion clinic in Pensacola, Florida by an antiabortion zealot. Several months later, another abortion provider was shot (though not seriously wounded) in Kansas, and during this same year, there were nearly two hundred reports of the "stalking" of abortion staff and their family members, at their workplaces, homes, churches, and schools. In 1994, tragedy again struck the abortion providing community. In the summer, John Britton – the physician who had taken over David Gunn's duties in Pensacola – was murdered, along with James Barrett, a retired air force colonel, who had been acting as his voluntary escort. And in late December of that year, Shannon Lowney and Leanne Nichols, receptionists at two different clinics in Brookline, Massachusetts, were killed, and several others wounded, when a gunman walked into their clinics and started shooting randomly.[6]

There is no question that the climate of violence surrounding abortion facilities, and especially the murders that have occurred, have had a chilling effect on abortion provision. But it is a mistake to overemphasize the role of the terrorist wing of the antiabortion movement in the current crisis. Due in large part to television news coverage, images of firebombings and screaming protesters surrounding a clinic have become so emblematic of the "abortion conflict" in the American consciousness that it is important to remember how relatively recent such incidents are. There were only a handful of violent incidents at abortion clinics in the years immediately following *Roe*, and bombings and arson attempts did not occur in substantial numbers until the mid-1980s;[7] initially, these violent incidents were almost all the work of individuals or small groups of abortion opponents, acting in isolation. It was not until 1987 and 1988 that elements within the antiabortion movement, frustrated by their inability to abolish abortion through conventional political means, entered an unusually militant, often violent phase and created such mass organizations as Operation Rescue and similar groups. Immediately thereafter, clinic blockades became commonplace. But the problems in abortion provision long predated this escalation in antiabortion intimidation. In the period immediately after the *Roe* decision in 1973 – some fifteen years *before* the emergence of groups like Operation Rescue – most U.S. medical institutions were refusing to acknowledge abortion as a legitimate component of women's health care. The majority of non-Catholic hospitals did not establish abortion services. In spite of the fact that abortion was quickly to become the most sought after elective surgery in the United States,[8] abortion training did not become a routine component of ob/gyn residencies. Thus, though the violence and intimidation associated with some of the opponents of abortion may explain why, in the 1990s, a particular community is without a clinic, it is not an adequate explanation of why – individual physicians' support notwithstanding – mainstream medicine has long distanced itself from abortion. I will suggest in the following chapters that it is the medical community itself, and not Operation Rescue, that bears chief responsibility for the present marginalization of abortion provision.

This book will convey the contested terrain of abortion provision through the eyes of a group of physicians whose experiences in the pre-*Roe* era convinced them of the necessity of safe abortion. Their involvement with abortion provision started when the procedure was still illegal and continued after the *Roe* decision. By focusing on the providers, my intention is to emphasize a seemingly obvious, yet largely undiscussed aspect of the abortion issue – that the actual delivery of abortions cannot take place unless some persons are willing to view this phenomenon as their "work." That is, in addition to all the other ways in which American culture approaches abortion – as a bitterly divisive political conflict, as a complex moral and ethical issue, as (depending on one's opinion) a symbol of contemporary women's aspirations for equality or of their selfishness – I argue that we must also understand abortion as an *occupation*. Once we think of abortion in this way, we are led to ask questions about abortion work that apply to all occupations – questions of motivation to perform this work, the gratifications and stresses associated with it, its relationship to other occupations, the importance of collegial affirmation, and so on.[9] This book pursues such questions about abortion work, focusing on the longstanding difficulties in the relationship between abortion provision and the larger field of medicine. The experiences – both before and after *Roe* – of the providers recounted here offer us a unique lens through which we can, on the one hand, better understand the current crisis in the availability of abortion, and, on the other, appreciate why, for some medical practitioners, there is no conscionable choice but to provide such services.

CHAPTER ONE

"I've Been Lucky to Have Been Part of This": Jane Hodgson and the Unending Struggle for Legal Abortion

In 1971, Jane Hodgson, a prominent obstetrician/gynecologist in St. Paul, Minnesota, became the only physician in United States history to be convicted of performing an abortion in a hospital.[1] Hodgson had performed this abortion openly, as a deliberate attempt to provoke a challenge to Minnesota's restrictive abortion policies. From the time of her test case to the present, Hodgson has committed herself to a career that includes both provision of abortions and activism on behalf of expanding abortion services. This dedication to the abortion issue has brought tremendous changes to Hodgson's life. A self-described "Eisenhower Republican" in the 1950s, she had achieved the pinnacle of medical respectability as president of the Minnesota Obstetrics/Gynecology Society; her association with abortion, however, ultimately caused her to become one of the most controversial medical figures in her state.

Though her willingness to serve as a test case – and thus put herself at considerable risk of imprisonment and loss of license – was quite unusual, in other respects, Hodgson's experiences are typical of those of a larger group of physicians who became involved, in various ways, with abortion provision in the years immediately preceding the landmark *Roe v. Wade* decision in 1973. An examination of Hodgson's personal history, therefore, will serve as an introduction to the key themes of this book: the mounting frustrations with anti-abortion regulations that led otherwise highly conventional physicians to various degrees of law breaking and law bending; the surprising irony that the legalization of abortion that occurred with *Roe* solved neither the problems of many women seeking abortions, nor of the physicians willing to provide them; and, finally, the profound ways physicians' lives are often transformed – at both the professional and personal levels – by their involvement with abortion.

Jane Hodgson was born in 1915 in rural Minnesota. She does not recall the abortion issue looming large in her childhood even though her father was a country doctor. The connection she does draw, however, between her early years and later abortion activity was the humanistic character of her father's medical practice, which she was able to observe as she accompanied him on his rounds. "He was as kind to the prostitutes in the county jail as he was to his private patients."

Hodgson graduated high school at the age of fifteen and then attended Carleton College. She was a medical student at the University of Minnesota in the 1930s and recalls her interest at that time in Margaret Sanger, "who was in and out of jail all the time because of her birth control activities." But in her medical school years at Minnesota and later in advanced obstetrical/gynecological training at the Mayo Clinic in the early 1940s, Hodgson received little training in abortion technique – and much antiabortion propaganda. "I had been taught in medical school that to invade the uterus was the most dangerous thing you could do. There are all kinds of complications. It was almost a superstition. We were also taught that it was illegal, and we saw all the criminal cases with those horrible infections, with some of them dying. You began to believe how dangerous it was. My whole experience, even at Mayo, we were never taught how to do a therapeutic abortion. . . . All we did was learn how to complete an abortion that had already been started. We always put a patient to sleep, it was a big deal."

Hodgson started a private practice in obstetrics and gynecology in the Twin Cities area in 1947, some twenty-six years before *Roe*. She quickly became successful. Besides a thriving practice, she embarked on research in a number of areas, achieving particular prominence with the innovation of a new form of early pregnancy test.[2] She was the recipient of a number of community service awards in this period, including the "I Care" award from the local Republican party. In 1964, she was elected president of the Minnesota Obstetrical/Gynecological Society.

Not surprisingly, as one of only a handful of female ob/gyns in practice in the Twin Cities area during that period, she was flooded with requests for abortions by her patients. "I saw more than my share of women who didn't want to be pregnant. . . . The tears that have been shed in my office in those days, you wouldn't believe." The hospitals in which Hodgson worked had a therapeutic abortion committee[3] but approved abortions only in the face of life-threatening conditions. Even some medically indicated abortions, seemingly beyond dispute, were difficult to get through the committee: "I remember one abortion I did that caused a lot of discussion – a young woman who had two sons; she had breast cancer that had metastasized, her life expectancy was short. She got pregnant from a diaphragm failure. It was a matter of increasing her life expectancy to interrupt that pregnancy. I remember how heartless some of those people were when we were discussing that case."

Like other physicians during the 1950s and 1960s, Hodgson had several strategies for dealing with unwanted pregnancies among her patients. In the 1950s, she made many referrals to "maternity homes" in the Midwest, institutions where young women would carry their pregnancies to term, put their babies up for adoption, and return to their communities with their "secret" intact.[4] By the 1960s, with the help of the local arm of the Clergy Consultation Service – a national organization that had been set up to help women and their physicians locate reliable abortion services – she was able to refer patients with resources to abortion providers outside the country and, shortly thereafter, to states with liberalized abortion policies.

These options were inadequate to handle the demand, however. It became increasingly clear to Hodgson that certain of her patients with unwanted pregnancies would seek out illegal abortions and thus were at medical risk. "I saw many different types of patients, for example, the frantic college student who didn't know where to turn, her future was going to be blasted if she continued her pregnancy. I knew that in spite of my advice, she would go out and find someone – there were all kinds of people doing abortions – and come back infected and bleeding. . . . I'd have to advise them from a health point of view not to have an abortion, to try and figure out some other solution, because the abortion would be such a risk."

The frustration that Hodgson felt about the risk to many of her own patients was compounded by the hypocrisy she perceived among many of her medical colleagues at that time. "Many of the physicians then who were publicly antiabortion, they would constantly be calling me if their wives or daughters had unplanned pregnancies, and of course, for *them*, I was supposed to get consultation and get it through [a therapeutic abortion committee], and everybody would look the other way. . . . The hypocrisy of it! Or they could afford to go to England or someplace and get it done. . . . It was a matter of different standards of medical care."

Throughout the 1950s and 1960s, Hodgson and her husband, Francis Quattlebaum, a cardiovascular surgeon, made periodic visits to medical facilities in the developing world, including several tours with Project Hope on a medical volunteer mission, which included both teaching and patient care. She credits this exposure to Third World poverty as a major force in sensitizing her to the importance of both fertility control and access to good medical care. "I became so conscious of the problems of the poor and the hungry – I didn't see that many hungry people here in Minnesota."

A visit to a Puerto Rican hospital during the 1950s, where she witnessed an open flouting of antiabortion laws, made a particularly strong impression on Hodgson. "Frank and I went and made rounds there, and this doctor took us around, he had his gold cross and was very Catholic. . . . I saw that they were scheduling many D. & C.'s* and tubal ligations. I asked him about that. 'Are these abortions that you do?' I can remember it so well. He was rather defensive, but said, 'When a woman has eight children, and she comes to me wanting an abortion, because she can't feed another one, I have to do it.' I was so impressed. I thought what a difference with our own state, because I

*"Dilation and curettage," an operation in which the cervix is opened and the lining of the uterus is scraped out, was commonly used for hospital-based abortions until the late 1960s, as well as for various other indications.

would see the same kind of patient at home, and I couldn't do anything, and here he was in a Catholic society."

Meanwhile, in her Minnesota private practice, Hodgson continued to be faced with patients with unwanted pregnancies. As she put
it, "It got very wearing to always be turning people down.... I got
tired of it." In her case, then, it was not–as it was for some others to
be discussed later–one particularly memorable case, but rather the
accumulation of experience that transformed her from someone
only mildly concerned with abortion to an abortion activist. It was
the combination of her patients' demands and the hypocrisy of her
physician colleagues; the results of botched abortions she saw in the
emergency rooms and the lack of compassion expressed by those on
her hospital's therapeutic abortion committee; the different options
available to rich and poor patients, and her observations in the developing world that led her to an intense period of thinking and studying
about abortion. "My position on abortion evolved. I had been taught
that abortion was immoral. I gradually came to change, I came to feel
that the law was immoral. There were all these young women whose
health was being ruined, whose lives were being ruined, whose
plans had to be changed. From my point of view, it was poor medicine, it was poor public health policy. After much soul searching, I realized that no other person could make that decision."

Hodgson became increasingly outspoken, within medical circles,
about the need to legalize abortion. In a strongly worded editorial,
published in *Minnesota Medicine* in 1970, she chided her colleagues
for their indifference to the fifty-two girls aged fourteen and under
who had recently been delivered of term pregnancies in that state.
Directly confronting the thorny issue of abortion and "reverence for
life," Hodgson wrote, "I am personally not concerned as to whether
life begins with the two-cell, four-cell, or eight-cell division but I *am*
extremely concerned with the quality of life that will result from the
division. We should be more concerned with the welfare of living
teenagers and women than with the future of a few embryonal
cells."[5] In a similar statement about pregnant teenagers, published
shortly thereafter in the same journal, Hodgson wrote of the "immorality" of "compulsory pregnancy" for poor teenagers, arguing that

the same options should exist for the underprivileged as for the daughters of physicians such as herself.[6]

This evolution in Hodgson's thinking about abortion eventually culminated in her decision in 1970 to openly challenge Minnesota's abortion law. Several years before, she had begun attending law school at night; although she was unable to finish because of illness, her two years of course work did familiarize her with the legal intricacies of abortion law both in Minnesota and nationally, and gave her some sense of what kind of legal strategy to pursue. Thus, by 1970 – some twenty-three years into her private practice – growing increasingly impatient with the obstructions of the hospital committee system for patients with medical indications for abortion, and frustrated by her utter inability to help patients who only had "social" indications for the procedure, Hodgson was, by her own admission, "subconsciously looking for a test case to challenge the law . . . and I had the perfect case walk into my office."

Hodgson's "perfect case" was a young woman in her twenties, Nancy Widmeyer. In Hodgson's view, she was highly suitable for a court challenge in several respects: medical, social, and personal. She had been diagnosed with rubella (German measles) in the fourth week of her pregnancy, a disease she contracted from her two children, who also had received this diagnosis from their pediatrician. Moreover, she was married and the mother of two. Thus, as Hodgson put it, "she wasn't single and she wouldn't offend anybody." Finally, in terms of personality, Widmeyer seemed ideal. "I explained to her that she could have gone out of state [by 1970, a number of states permitted abortion in cases of rubella, because of the likelihood of deformity], or I could have taken her through the hospital consultation [therapeutic abortion committee] system, but I told her that very few people would get through that system and there was a great need to demonstrate to the people of Minnesota how horrible our law was, and would she be willing to go to court, if necessary. She was a brave gal, she had a sense of justice. She said, 'Why should I have to go away to have this done? I want you to do it, here.' "

Hodgson's first step after securing the cooperation of this patient was to go to federal court in Minnesota and ask that the current abortion law be overturned. When this request was ultimately turned down, she went ahead and scheduled Widmeyer for a D. & C. in St. Paul-Ramsey Hospital. As Hodgson had anticipated, the police were notified and, shortly after the procedure, came to her office and arrested her. "I had to go down to the jail and get fingerprinted. . . . I was a little shocked seeing all the characters down there. I hadn't been down to the police department in quite a while."

The arrest set off a three-year period of legal activity, during which Hodgson's license to practice medicine in Minnesota was in question. After an initial conviction – making her the first physician in U.S. history to be convicted for performing an abortion in a hospital – she appealed to the Minnesota Supreme Court; while this appeal was still in progress, the U.S. Supreme Court handed down the *Roe v. Wade* decision, thus overturning her earlier conviction.

Hodgson became highly visible in the Twin Cities area immediately before the abortion (when news of her request to the federal court was prominent in local media) and especially after the abortion, when she was arrested and went to trial. This period brought enormous changes to Hodgson's life, at all levels, and was her first introduction to the intensity and polarization of the abortion debate.

Hodgson had not previously thought of herself as an "activist." "It's not in my nature to lead a movement, I'm not the kind to get up on soapboxes." She nonetheless came to be a focal point for activists on both sides of the abortion issue. Supporters in St. Paul, to her pleased surprise, started the Dr. Jane Hodgson Defense Fund to pay for her legal expenses. She began to get many phone calls from both out-of-town supporters and opponents. Some of the supportive phone calls, however, cautioned her against the actions she was taking. "I was getting these phone calls from doctors who had tried similar things. There was one man down in Iowa, I don't remember his name, and he said, 'It's not worth it; I've done the same thing and I've lost all my practice. . . . It's a disaster, you can't lick this thing, don't do it.'" An early and quite painful indication of the price she was to pay for taking such a stand was the abrupt resignation of Hodgson's longtime office nurse. "She was my favorite nurse. I had delivered all her kids. . . . She left the day I did that abortion in the hospital and I haven't seen her since."

Predictably, the 1971 trial itself showcased the deep divisions within the medical community at that time over the abortion issue. Hodgson's lawyer was Roy Lucas, a brilliant young lawyer based in New York, who simultaneously was influential in developing the legal strategy in the *Roe v. Wade* case.[7] Testifying on behalf of Hodgson were various nationally known figures, including the late Christopher Tietze, an eminent biostatician and one of the leading scholars of the public health dimensions of abortion.[8] Hodgson recalls Tietze's participation in the trial as a particular boost for her. "Chris came out with his beret and turtleneck. Kind of shook things up. Everyone thought he was a traveling witness for pay. The state's attorney was trying to get him to admit that he was being paid a big sum to come out here and testify. 'Is it true, Dr. Tietze, that you have testified in a number of other cases?' 'Oh yes, many.' 'Have you accepted any money for any of your testimony?' 'No, I didn't.' 'What is your fee in this case?' 'Nothing.' 'Well then, why are you here?' And he very quietly said – he could never get ruffled – 'For the sake of justice.' Everybody just smiled."

John McKelvey, then the chairman of the department of obstetrics and gynecology at the University of Minnesota and an ardent anti-abortionist, was a key witness for the state. "He came over and he brought all his residents with him – I guess he wanted them to see what happens if you take the wrong path. He testified that it was wholly unnecessary to abort a woman that had rubella, that it should never be done, how terribly dangerous a procedure it was.... He tried to present some out-of-date materials – very poor work – that showed the low incidence of deformities from rubella." Lucas was able to refute McKelvey's findings with other publications, and furthermore, through copious research the lawyer discovered instances of plagiarism in McKelvey's own writings. "Roy brought that out, and McKelvey was just furious, sputtering, and he left. Never spoke to me again, the rest of his life. He's dead now. But I would run into him frequently, and he would just never speak to me."

In spite of the strong support Hodgson received from many influential individuals within medicine, she was particularly disappointed by the lack of any support from organized medicine, especially the American College of Obstetricians and Gynecologists. In one of the few moments of bitterness that Hodgson allowed herself in the course of many hours of interviews, she said, in response to my question of what the ACOG had done to help her case, "*Nothing*, not a thing. They never did anything." By coincidence, a regional section of ACOG was holding its annual meeting in St. Paul at the time of the trial – literally across the street from the courthouse – and Lucas suggested that Hodgson ask one of the national officers of the College to come and testify on behalf of abortion reform. This request was refused. "It wasn't a matter of his time schedule or anything like that, he just plain didn't think it was the political thing to do. I wasn't asking him to testify *for me*, but to testify about the need for a medical service being provided." The Minnesota Obstetrical/Gynecological Society (of which Hodgson had previously been president) was at that time dominated by an antiabortion leadership and took a stand opposing Hodgson, further contributing to her growing awareness of the polarization created by her case.

On the other hand, Hodgson received outspoken support from many medical students at the University of Minnesota, who were becoming deeply interested in abortion politics at that time. To her special satisfaction, she also received many indications of support from physicians at the Mayo Clinic, where she had years earlier received advanced training. "They asked me to write an article [on abortion] for their alumni journal, and they reprinted many copies of it and used it for propaganda purposes, and the doctors there came up and testified. The support I got there – it was almost unanimous."[9]

When Hodgson first made the decision to challenge her state's abortion law, she was well aware that she was risking both a jail sentence and her career. When asked to explain how she could have contemplated jeopardizing so much, Hodgson was, first, philosophical. "I was in the right spot at the right time. It was just something I couldn't avoid. It just seemed like a role that had been created for me and it was sort of inevitable, kind of a role you feel you have to play."

When pressed further to recollect her feelings at the time she was risking a jail sentence (estimated by her lawyer to be about four years), Hodgson answered initially in quite stoic terms. "I figured I was fifty-five and I'd led a very good life. I'd been sheltered financially, really, and I had male support – first my father, and then my husband. . . . I felt I'd had a very good life, so what if it's over? I'd had good health, no real troubles. I'd been blessed. I'd had fifty-five years, how many can you expect? . . . I was ready to go to jail, and I thought, 'Well, I'll write a book.' "

As this conversation progressed, however, Hodgson acknowledged that the action she took in performing an illegal abortion was sharply at odds with her apolitical, conventional upbringing – "we always conformed to society" – and with the image she had cultivated as a successful physician in private practice – "I guess I always tried to have people think well of me. In practice you have to." In contrast to the stoicism expressed earlier, she also revealed the enormous personal cost that the loss of her medical license would have entailed. "That was hard to visualize, because it had been my whole life. It was something I had worked very hard to get, back in the days when I went to med school – it was very hard for women, at that point, to get advanced training, to get your Boards – all of which I had by 1947. Even now, when I'm in semiretirement, slowing down, I miss it terribly, and I haven't quit of course, I refuse to retire. Because it's your whole life. . . . I think medicine has been my religion probably."

There is, of course, no one simple answer as to why certain individuals, such as Hodgson, decide to risk so much to act upon matters of principle. Hodgson, when pressed to reflect on her perseverance during that period, several times acknowledged her own "stubbornness" in the face of a struggle whose favorable outcome she had come to see as "a real necessity, something that has got to be done." Beyond that, she gave a suggestive portrait of someone who, in midlife, came to discover a profoundly political aspect within herself. "People get wrapped up in causes, I guess – and I must admit that I did. It was the matter of establishing the truth on an issue."

The period after Hodgson's conviction and during her appeal before the Minnesota Supreme Court was a highly stressful one. She found herself professionally at a standstill, reluctant to practice obstetrics in her home state because of the uncertainty of the outcome of her appeal, and she became demoralized as the appeal dragged on. "The Court would announce its decisions on Fridays, and it got so depressing each Friday, when I'd realize I'd have to wait another week to find out." Thus, when she was invited to become medical director of the recently opened Preterm clinic in Washington, D.C. (Washington by 1971 had legalized abortion and Preterm was among the first freestanding abortion clinics in the country), she saw it as a welcome escape from the stress of her legal struggles in Minnesota. She worked as Preterm's medical director for several years, flying back to her family in St. Paul on weekends.

Professionally, the Preterm experience was highly gratifying, *albeit* challenging. "We did about sixty abortions a day. It was a wonderful service, and women were coming from all over the United States where it was illegal. They traveled long distances. . . . And then the problem of getting care for them after they'd go home. They'd call up and be in trouble and we didn't know where to send them. There were no doctors to take care of them. It was quite an experience."

Directing the Preterm clinic also gave Hodgson the opportunity to initiate ground-breaking research on outpatient abortion procedures in a normal population. She collaborated on a study of the use of antibiotics after outpatient abortion, which helped to establish standard procedures for the many abortion clinics that in a few years would be established across the country. She wrote papers on complication rates, which turned out to be remarkably low. "I reported twenty thousand consecutive abortions with a complication rate of 0.9 percent. We had no deaths.[10] Back in the early days, the clinic had an ambulance that was kept on hand all the time. It was rarely, if ever, used and finally they got rid of it. It just fell apart from no use but we didn't know if it might be necessary if a woman started bleeding in the clinic and we had to rush her to the hospital."

When asked if the low complication rates were surprising to her, she replied, "Oh, yes, because it was contrary to everything that had been taught, and I felt it was very important to write about it. I did a lot of writing letters to editors. Some of the pro-life doctors would write articles about the high infection rate – maybe, anecdotal, they'd see one or two bad cases and say how terrible it was, our doing abortions in Washington. In fact there was an article that appeared here in Minnesota, one that I had to counter."[11]

Making the adjustment to the Preterm model – which was characterized by a "team approach" and a decidedly nonhierarchal ethos – was admittedly difficult for Hodgson, as it was for many of the physicians who worked in the first generation of freestanding abortion clinics. "I'd never worked in a clinic. I'd always had my own private practice and run my own show. I was not accustomed to counselors participating in medical decisions. It was a team approach that was entirely new to me and not easy, I might add. . . . They had music playing all the time during procedures, very casual, no uniforms [on staff]. I was accustomed to operating in a very serious room with caps and gowns and masks and scrubbing for every procedure and to suddenly go in and there'd be a patient up in stirrups with no drape. . . . It was a shocker. And I thought, we're bound to have some calamities, we're going to have some accidents, it's just bound to happen. And it was just like walking on eggshells. But I gradually learned and gained my confidence."

In January 1973, after she had been at Preterm approximately two years, the *Roe* decision was announced, which implied that Hodgson's conviction by the Minnesota court was overruled, and that she was able once again to practice in her home state. Though during this period Hodgson still had one teenage daughter living at home (the other was in college), and her colleagues at Preterm made it clear that she was free to leave immediately if she wished, Hodgson chose to stay in Washington for several additional months, a decision she made for both symbolic and practical reasons. "I thought that [delaying her return] was kind of important, realizing that if I came tearing right back that would minimize the importance of what I'd been doing. . . . I said, 'No, I want to finish this.' " Besides wanting to finish the various research projects in which she was engaged, Hodgson also valued the political opportunities inherent in being the medical director of one of the preeminent freestanding abortion clinics in the country. "I hated to relinquish the platform of medical director of Preterm because I did a lot of correspondence about all this, I was doing a lot of public speaking." With the encouragement of her family, Hodgson remained in Washington until the fall of 1973.

After Hodgson returned to St. Paul, she immediately embarked on a series of activities that was to make her the most visible abortion activist within the medical community in the state. In spite of the animosity of the chair of obstetrics and gynecology at the University of Minnesota medical school, she became a member of the clinical faculty at the school, and in that capacity headed up the fertility control clinic at St. Paul-Ramsey Hospital. "They needed somebody just to keep up with the demand for abortion services, and the doctors – none of them knew how to do them – and they really needed me to provide the service. After all, it was legal." She also for a time became medical director of the newly established abortion clinic of Planned Parenthood of Minnesota, as well as the director of the Midwest Health Clinic for Women, a private nonprofit freestanding abortion facility based in Minneapolis. Hodgson also began to strategize how to give women in outlying areas access to abortion services. "My great aim then was to establish some outpatient clinics in the state of Minnesota so that the people wouldn't have to come so far. You know, the distances are so great, and there was no place else in the state where they were providing the service, so I wanted to get up to Duluth, and get one established up there, and we were also thinking about Rochester. That fell through, however, but we did get a good clinic established in Duluth. We did about one hundred procedures a month up there, and the women came from Canada and all along the North Shore, very worthwhile. So for a while there I was running three clinics, which was a big job."

After her return to Minnesota, Hodgson also continued the legal activism that she had first undertaken with her 1970 trial. She sued one of the hospitals at which she had staff privileges because the institution had not taken steps to establish an abortion service after *Roe.* "Obviously I wasn't very popular with the hospital at that time." Disturbed by what she had seen throughout her career of "the two standards of medicine," in which the poor do not have the same care as the nonpoor, she joined in legal actions, in Minnesota and beyond, concerning subsidized abortions for Medicaid recipients. "I was very concerned about the poor women during that period. All the time I was at Ramsey, we'd see these women who could not afford a second trimester abortion because there was no money available to pay for it, and these women couldn't afford it." Hodgson testified as an expert witness in the *McCrae v. Harris* case, a Supreme Court case in which the Court upheld the banning of the use of federal monies for abortions for poor women. She was also deeply involved in litigation concerning parental notification laws and abortion, and was the lead plaintiff in *Hodgson v. Minnesota*, the 1990 Supreme Court case which stipulated that a state may require a teenage girl to notify both parents before obtaining an abortion, as long as the law provides the alternative of a judicial hearing.[12]

Since 1973 Hodgson has also been very active as an expert witness throughout the United States on behalf of various abortion providers charged in malpractice cases. Her periodic testimony in various Canadian courts on behalf of Henry Morgentaler–the leading medical crusader for abortion rights in Canada–has been especially gratifying to her, both because of her admiration of Morgentaler and because of the opportunity to influence abortion policy in another country. "I think perhaps the thing I've enjoyed most in court was going to Canada in the Morgentaler cases. . . . I have been up there three times now because they try to keep putting him back in jail. To be able to educate another country is rather special . . . you feel like you're really maybe doing something, and I was able to point out to them, the last time, the number of Canadian women who had come over to our Duluth clinic, and what the experiences of these Canadian women were, and how they had to leave the country. That was very effective testimony. So I kept a record of a couple hundred or so patients and their stories, and I related them all day up there. . . . I went up to Newfoundland and gave a paper on abortion way back in 1971 or 1972, when it was strictly illegal there and it made Newfoundland headlines, and everyone was real shocked that I would come in and talk openly about a thing like that. . . . That's kind of gratifying when you go in a country where women have no abortion rights at all and you at least get them talking about it. I got the paper published in the Canadian health journal so I think maybe I have helped Canada. So these things along the way make it worthwhile."[13]

The polarization of her professional and social circles that Hodgson first experienced at the time of her 1970 trial intensified after her return to Minnesota in 1973. When she resumed private practice, certain old patients did not return to her – "though new ones did. . . . I always had more than I could do, it was always very busy. Maybe there was some financial loss but that wasn't that important to me." More upsetting to Hodgson was the evident transformation in her collegial networks. This became very clear to her, shortly after her return, when she received a stony reception from peers at the annual meeting of the Minnesota Obstetrical/Gynecological Society, an organization which she had once served as president. "That was really a contrast, having been president and involved in all their politics, and I came back from Washington and gave a paper on abortion complications at the state meeting – but the whole atmosphere of friendliness was gone totally. Although there were obvious exceptions, doctors who were longtime friends."

Hodgson's career, in the twenty-odd years from 1973 through the early 1990s, has similarly been marked by various skirmishes – some petty, some more substantial – with antiabortion forces within the medical community. For example, while on a medical teaching visit in China, she received a letter notifying her that her status as a clinical faculty member at the University of Minnesota was being terminated. "They claimed I hadn't fulfilled my requirements of teaching, and actually I had more than done it at St. Paul-Ramsey. It was a matter of the records getting screwed up. I do think it was politically motivated because the doctor that was responsible was very active in the pro-life movement. . . . I think if I had not been involved in [abortion], this never would have happened. Because I have never had any reason for anyone to attack my credentials, I have never had a lawsuit." After her return, Hodgson arranged for her reinstatement. "It was for the principle of the thing, because I would appear in court somewhere and didn't want to lose my associate professorship." Similarly, while maintaining a very active publishing record in the years since 1973, Hodgson has periodically encountered resistance to her work on the part of editors or reviewers which she defines as "political" rather than legitimately "academic."

In personal terms, one of the most painful costs of abortion involvement came when Hodgson attended her fiftieth reunion at Carleton College. "They were giving me an alumni award at that re-

union. I learned later from the committee that it was a very hot discussion whether they should give it to me or not but they finally did.
But I remember it was very painful. I don't usually go to reunions. I
hate them. I hadn't been to one and some of these people I hadn't seen
since college, and I'd rush forward to greet them and they'd turn
away. It was kind of a low blow and I think that bothered me maybe
as much as anything."

Upsetting as such incidents have been, Hodgson is unequivocal in
her view that the transformations in her professional and social network as a result of her stand on abortion have on balance been positive ones. Reflecting on the changes brought about by her initial decision to challenge Minnesota law, she said, "It was a total surprise and
kind of shakeup in your friends and support. People that you never
expected would come forth and be so great and you made new
friends, and other people that you had thought were good friends . . .
amazing what you find out in a situation like that." Hodgson is also
aware of what the professional tradeoffs have been because of her
abortion stance and here, too, she feels she has "gained far more than
I have lost." While her abortion activism has obviously closed some
doors – in certain Minnesota medical circles Hodgson perceives herself as "controversial and untouchable" – it has opened others, especially to national medical and legal arms of the reproductive freedom
movement. "The people I've known who are involved in this issue are
on the whole more interesting to me – I've made friends I never would
have made."

In this light, an especially meaningful moment for Hodgson was a
meeting with Harry Blackmun, the Supreme Court justice who au-
thored the *Roe* decision. This visit took place shortly after the historic
decision was handed down, and the two were able to discuss their
similar experiences of extreme visibility on the abortion issue. "He'd
been aware of my case, because he was from Minnesota and would
come back regularly to visit. I went to see him, he was kind of like an
idol of mine. . . . He told me how much mail he'd been getting over
this thing, and how much soul searching he had done. . . . He truly is
a man of courage. That [visit] was about as satisfying as anything. I
felt like I was truly relating and he truly understood."

The twenty-odd years since Hodgson returned to Minnesota from

Washington, then, have been marked by her continual legal battles against abortion restrictions and a growing estrangement from the medical establishment, in Minnesota and beyond. The initial disillusionment she felt at the time of her 1970 trial, when ACOG failed to give her official support, has continued in the years after *Roe.* In the early 1980s, in a major text she edited on abortion, Hodgson wrote about the freestanding clinic model with which she was so deeply involved: "What does the future hold for this new phenomenon in our health care system? Will hospitals eventually absorb these clinics in the same way that they are attaching outpatient mini-surgical clinics to their institutions? Will the medical schools absorb or grant affiliation to any of the four hundred clinics now operating in the United States? . . . It is only by academic affiliation that proper standards of medical service, education, and research will be continuously defined. Academic affiliation is also a prerequisite to the provision of sufficient numbers of doctors for this new subspecialty."[14]

As this book will discuss, Hodgson's vision for the mainstreaming of abortion services into U.S. medical institutions has not been realized, save for occasional exceptions, and this failure on the part of medicine in general – and the field of obstetrics and gynecology in particular – is Hodgson's greatest disappointment. She is deeply concerned about the low numbers of doctors willing to provide abortion and colleagues' reactions to providers: "So many doctors scorn any other doctor who does abortion." She similarly expresses frustration with the lack of abortion training in ob/gyn residencies and the near-absolute omission of abortion-related topics from the annual meetings of ACOG.

Hodgson's transformation from a conventionally successful private practitioner in obstetrics/gynecology to one of the most visible physician advocates for abortion in the United States has, inevitably, led her to rethink earlier assumptions about mainstream medicine and her place within it. "I think frankly I've gotten turned off to the medical profession and organized medicine. I've been a maverick, and as the years go by I get more and more turned off by their decision making, and I haven't wanted to be involved in their politics. I've just gone in a different direction. Originally, I wanted respectability and wanted to get to the top medically, and politically too, when I got out of med school, but I came to realize that's not for me. I don't admire organized medicine for many reasons – doctors have become too greedy, and many of them are too narrow in their perspective."

An additional political transformation brought about by Hodgson's experiences with the abortion struggle is her growing acknowledgment of a "feminist" sensibility. This has come after an earlier period in which she had felt quite removed from the women's movement that had reemerged in the United States in the late 1960s and early 1970s. When asked if her initial decision to perform the unauthorized abortion had been informed by an identification with feminism, Hodgson replied: "No, it wasn't. I really think I was truly a feminist, but I never was active in the cause particularly, and I'd been critical of them. I think they made a lot of mistakes in the movement. . . . Criticism of the male, for instance, and male physicians. I think a lot of the stands they took – I really didn't quite understand. [In 1970], I really didn't associate myself in particular."

For Hodgson, an acceptance of a "feminist" identity became persuasive when she came to reflect on the inseparability of feminism and reproductive freedom. "In retrospect, I think that reproductive freedom is the most important issue of the movement. I don't think it ever would have been achieved without birth control pills in the 1960s. Just from seeing it in my office, seeing how women became self-sufficient and independent because they could control their reproduction. Before 1960, when they didn't have anything but a lousy diaphragm, women were helpless creatures. They were just victims of circumstances, so many of them. They'd come in, I'd have to wipe off the tears. And then, when they began to get [better contraception] you could just see them getting into jobs, planning their lives, and I think that, plus the legalization of abortion, when contraceptives failed, has been the biggest factor in the feminist movement. . . . I think it [reproductive freedom] will be considered one of the biggest issues, the most important movement of this century. Somebody compared it to the discovery of fire."

In her late seventies, in "semiretirement," Jane Hodgson continues to teach and care for patients in the developing world. She has re-

cently worked in a school-based clinic in St. Paul, offering contraceptive services to teenagers. She is involved in various legal cases
concerning abortion provision; an especially gratifying victory was
a recent case, in which she served as a lead plaintiff, that restored
Medicaid funding of abortions in Minnesota. She writes and lectures
on a broad range of issues concerning reproductive health. She also
still performs abortions. The Duluth Women's Health Center, which
she helped found, is unable to recruit any local physicians to work
there, so Hodgson for several years has been among a number of physicians who fly in from out of town to work at the clinic.[15]

Despite the many setbacks the abortion movement has suffered
since 1973, Hodgson retains a stubborn optimism about the future.
"I'm resigned really to this slow pace, but I think inevitably women
will have the full right to abortion. It will be a major step forward."
A major source of her optimism is her ongoing contact with young
medical students. Interaction with these students reassures her that,
as her cohort nears retirement, there is a replacement generation of
abortion providers in the pipeline. She drew particularly sweet satisfaction, when meeting with a group of pro-choice medical students,
to learn that one of the young women present was the daughter of a
former state official who years earlier had sparred with Hodgson in
court over abortion restrictions. "It's a complete cycle. Here her father was, on the other side, restricting Medicaid payments and everything else, and now his own daughter . . . it makes you feel good."

Notwithstanding the considerable professional and personal
costs, Jane Hodgson expresses no regrets about the path on which
she embarked in 1970 when she decided to openly perform an illegal
abortion. "I think in many ways I've been lucky to have been part of
this. I mean life is dull if you can't get involved in something worthwhile. If I hadn't gotten involved, I would have gone through life
probably being perfectly satisfied to go to the medical society parties
and it would have been very, very dull. I would have been bored silly."

CHAPTER TWO

U.S. Medicine
and the Marginalization of Abortion

The relationship of organized medicine and abortion in the United States has always been marked by strain and ambivalence. What emerges from an overview of this relationship, from the nineteenth century through the *Roe* era, is a portrait of a profession increasingly splintered. While dominant medical organizations have at times taken strong stands against legal abortion, and at other times been conspicuous for their silence, other segments of the profession – notably progressive factions within obstetrics and gynecology and public health – have found their colleagues' antiabortion stands to be untenable and have worked assiduously for acceptance of abortion within medical circles. The point of this chapter is to convey the cross pressures about the abortion issue that individual physicians in practice and training – such as the subjects of this book – felt in the years leading up to *Roe*.

THE ANTIABORTION CAMPAIGN OF THE AMERICAN MEDICAL ASSOCIATION

Until the middle of the nineteenth century, abortion was only minimally regulated in the United States. The prevailing standard was that abortions that occurred before "quickening" (which generally occurs between the fourth and sixth months of pregnancy) were not regulated at all, and there was minimal attempt to police abortions that occurred afterward. Abortion apparently was commonly practiced, and abortion services were freely advertised in newspapers, offered by practitioners of widely varying degrees of medical training and credentials. Much of the abortion activity of the period consisted of women's attempts to give themselves abortions using various herbs and drugs, which they either purchased from an apothecary or ordered through the mail. The drive to criminalize abortion, which started in mid-century and peaked by the early 1880s, when all the states had enacted antiabortion statutes, stemmed from a variety of motivations, including societal anxiety about the declining birth rates of Anglo-Saxon women in comparison to those of newly arriving immigrants. The Roman Catholic church and many Protestant clergy, which up to this point had been silent on the abortion question, also participated in the campaign.

But as recent scholarship has demonstrated, the most important force in the campaign to criminalize abortion were the physicians.[1] The American Medical Association (AMA), founded in 1847, made the abortion struggle one of its highest priorities. The argument of these physicians, in brief, was that abortion was both an immoral act and a medically dangerous one, given the incompetence of many of the practitioners then. The abortion campaign of the nineteenth century thus is most usefully understood as a key component of a larger battle then under way: the attempt of "regular" or "elite" physicians (that is, those who were university-trained) to attain professional dominance over the wide range of "irregular" medical practitioners—healers, homeopaths, and the like—who had flourished throughout the first part of the nineteenth century. Abortion was a particularly fruitful territory over which to stake claims of professional monopoly, both because so much of the irregulars' activity was apparently abortion-based and because much abortion work was being done by laypeople with no claims whatsoever to medical credentials.[2]

The objective of regular physicians was not simply to abolish all abortions, however. Rather, the AMA argument, which ultimately prevailed, was that physicians should control the terms under which "approved" abortions were performed—that is, "legal" abortions were now to be confined to those performed in a hospital, for "medically indicated" reasons.

As with virtually all social conflicts over reproductive matters,[3] the nineteenth century AMA campaign against abortion contained an explicit dimension of gender politics. The arguments used then by many of the antiabortion physicians prefigure in many instances the rhetoric of the antiabortion movement of the present time: abortion represents a threat to male authority and the "traditional role" of women; abortion is a symbol of uncontrolled female sexuality, and an "unnatural" act. Above all, the aborting woman is selfish and self-indulgent. As the authors of the AMA's Committee on Criminal Abortion wrote in 1871 about this woman:

> She becomes unmindful of the course marked out for her by Providence, she overlooks the duties imposed on her by the marriage contract. She yields to the pleasures – but shrinks from the pains and responsibilities of maternity; and, destitute of all delicacy and refinement, resigns herself, body and soul, into the hands of unscrupulous and wicked men. Let not the husband of such a wife flatter himself that he possesses her affection. Nor can she in turn ever merit even the respect of a virtuous husband. She sinks into old age like a withered tree, stripped of its foliage; with the stain of blood upon her soul, she dies without the hand of affection to smooth her pillow.[4]

One well-known result of the "century of criminalization" that resulted from the efforts of the AMA was a flourishing market in illegal abortion. In addition to the abortions women attempted to give themselves, illegal abortions were done by nurses and midwives, lay abortionists, and physicians. A study published by Frederick Taussig in 1936 estimated a half-million illegal abortions were taking place in the United States annually; the Kinsey Report in 1953 suggested that nine out of ten premarital pregnancies among its respondents were aborted, while over 20 percent of the married women in the sample reported having had an abortion while married.[5] As already noted, estimates of illegal abortion in the 1950s and in the years immediately leading up to *Roe* range as high as 1.2 million per year.

This highly erratic system of illegal abortion inevitably carried with it a high degree of medical risk and of patient exploitation. Anywhere from one thousand to five thousand women per year are estimated to have died from illegal abortions in the pre-*Roe* era and

many thousands more were injured.[6] Moreover, the accounts of
women who obtained illegal abortions in that era often describe in-
tolerable situations:

> "More than the incredible filth of the place, and my fear on seeing it;
> more than the fear that I would surely become infected; more than the
> fact that the man was an alcoholic, and was drinking throughout the
> procedure – a whiskey glass in one hand, and a sharp instrument in the
> other; more than the indescribable pain, the most intense pain I have
> ever been subjected to; more than the humiliation of being told, 'You can
> take your pants down now, but you shoulda' – ha!ha! – kept them on
> before'; more than the degradation of being asked to perform a deviant
> sex act after he had aborted me . . . more than the hemorrhaging and the
> peritonitis and the hospitalization that followed; more even than the
> gut-twisting fear of being 'found out' and locked away for perhaps 20
> years; more than all these things, those pitchy stairs and that dank, dark
> hallway and the door at the end of it stay with me and chill my blood
> still."[7]

> "Preparations for doing this were very complicated and anxiety-filled. I
> had to stand on a street corner in Washington, D.C., holding a copy of
> *Time* magazine. A woman was supposed to approach me and ask if I had
> a problem. . . . The next stage happened a week later. I was picked up by
> a car . . . by someone who took me to a place where there was a long
> black limousine waiting. . . . We left Washington, and the car stopped,
> and the driver said, 'And now, for fun, we're going to put these little gog-
> gles over your eyes.' . . . And then we arrived at a farmhouse. . . . There
> were guards standing around with guns. . . . I just remember being
> terrified."[8]

As with other illegal activities, some portion of the underground
abortion market inevitably involved police payoffs and connections
with organized crime. One police account in the early 1960s estimated that criminal abortion was the "third biggest racket" in the
United States, ranking only behind gambling and narcotics.[9]

LEGAL UNCERTAINTY, MEDICAL TURMOIL

For many doctors in practice in the years leading up to *Roe*, the criminalization of abortion created a highly frustrating system of legal and

medical confusion. It was a system, to repeat, in which all abortions were illegal except those "medically approved" abortions which took place in hospitals. Thus, the various providers, including physicians, who were performing the approximate million or so illegal abortions per year were theoretically risking arrest. With the benefit of historical hindsight, we now know that the majority of them were not prosecuted, and that many of those prosecuted were not ultimately convicted. The fairly low rates of prosecution and conviction can be explained by such factors as the police payoffs that were a significant aspect of many illegal abortion operations; the apparent sympathy of juries to the accused abortionist in a number of well known cases, which gave pause to district attorneys contemplating such prosecutions; and most generally, the secrecy to which all parties to the illegal abortion were committed.[10]

But my task here is not to assess the objective risk under which illegal abortionists operated, but rather to attempt to recapture the physicians' *perception* of risk in the pre-*Roe* era, such as the conscience physicians interviewed for this book, who were developing sympathy to women seeking abortions. For those in practice at this time, how risky did becoming involved in abortion seem? Here, as in so much else of the abortion story before *Roe*, there were enormous variations from place to place, and even abrupt changes within the same hospital, city, or state, according to changing political circumstances. For example, a situation where illegal abortions had been done with relative impunity could change quickly if a police chief was ordered to "clean up" a part of town where abortions were known to take place,[11] or a district attorney made the calculation that an antiabortion crusade would be politically beneficial to him. While most of the arrests that did take place were of lay abortionists, rather than physicians, periodic arrests of physicians did occur – most likely, if a patient had died, but occasionally on other grounds as well. Even if these arrests did not always lead to a conviction, the attendant publicity could be devastating to the physician's reputation. And even if a physician did not ultimately have to face a prison cell, the prospect of losing one's license to practice, which also was an outcome of some prosecutions, was very chilling to those considering performing abortions.

The presence of police in the wards of city hospitals, where many women who had had illegal abortions ended up, also reinforced the criminality of abortion in the minds of young practitioners. The amount of police surveillance varied from place to place, and across time periods, within the same place. In a number of states, such as New York, physicians were required by law to report a suspected illegal abortion, which would bring officers directly to the ward to question the patient.[12] The sight of police interrogating very sick patients, attempting to elicit from them the name of their abortionist, was particularly jarring to many young physicians.

But perhaps the most troubling aspect of the legal climate before *Roe* was the tremendous uncertainty under which even "legal" abortions took place. To recapitulate, when states banned abortions in the late nineteenth century, there were, in all instances, provisions for abortions "to save the life of the mother." Some states moreover passed vaguer statutes to preserve the "health," and eventually in some states, the "mental health" of the mother. But given the subjective judgments called for in many of these cases – how, precisely, does one define threats to the physical or mental health of the mother? – physicians felt themselves operating in a gray area between illegality and legality, not knowing if their judgments would be called into question by the legal system, or by fellow physicians with different attitudes toward abortion. The performance of abortions for reasons of suspected damage to the fetus, a practice that became increasingly common in the 1960s, brought further ambiguity to the issue of what constituted a "legal" abortion.

The celebrated cases of Sherri Finkbine in 1962 and the "San Francisco Nine" in 1966 illustrate the uncertainty of legal abortion in the pre-*Roe* era. In the former case, a Phoenix woman, pregnant with her fifth child, learned that the thalidomide drug her husband brought back from Europe for her to use as a sleeping pill was strongly associated with severe birth defects. Her physician arranged an abortion for her in a local hospital, but when news of the impending abortion became public, nervous hospital authorities cancelled the procedure, on the grounds that Arizona law permitted an abortion only to save the life of the mother. Ultimately Finkbine arranged to have an abortion in Sweden.[13]

In the second case, nine highly respected obstetricians/gynecologists in San Francisco were abruptly threatened with the loss of their licenses because they had been performing hospital-based abortions on women infected with rubella, a practice that was increasingly common in a number of states by the 1960s, as evidence of the link between this disease and birth defects became known. (Between 1962 and 1965, some fifteen thousand babies were born with defects attributed to a rubella epidemic.) The sudden decision to prosecute these physicians apparently was instigated by one individual, a strongly antiabortion member of the California Board of Medical Examiners. The case drew national media attention and an unprecedented show of support from influential physicians across the country; more than one hundred deans of medical schools protested this prosecution.[14] Ultimately, the charges against these physicians were dropped. Each of these cases was instrumental in mobilizing support for abortion reform in the 1960s: the Finkbine case among the public at large, and the San Francisco Nine within the medical community.

As the above events suggest, the medical climate with respect to abortion provision was increasingly in turmoil between 1940 and 1970. Most physicians – even in obstetrical/gynecological residencies – were not routinely taught how to perform abortions *per se* as part of their medical training. They were, however, taught the dilation and curettage technique, D. & C's. This technique – the major method for both illegal and legal abortions through the late 1960s – was also used for other gynecological procedures. Physicians who would be called upon to complete a "spontaneous abortion," i.e., a miscarriage, would be expected to use the D. & C. method. Similarly, if performing a sanctioned hospital abortion, ob/gyns would use the D. & C. method with the patient under general anesthesia.

But if they received only scanty training in the techniques of abortion, some physicians in this period apparently received ample antiabortion ideology as part of their training. When the subjects of this book were asked to recall what messages about abortion they had received in medical school and residency, one participant remembered that "antiabortion messages were given like a broken record – you can't violate the Hippocratic oath." Another remembered her medical school professor's reaction to a patient on the ward who had tried to abort herself using potassium permanganate tablets (highly corrosive tablets widely used to induce vaginal bleeding and thus to simulate a miscarriage). "She was bleeding heavily from her vagina because it had broken through to a blood vessel but she was not unconscious. And the attending doctor just said, 'This is a terrible thing to have done and you should be extremely ashamed of yourself.' So he was both condemning the patient and condemning the act to the medical student. Just all around negativity and no understanding of her plight." Others remembered silence not only about abortion but on all matters pertaining to sexuality. As a woman in medical school in the 1940s recounted, "We had one lecture on sex – for an hour – and that lecture was delivered by an outsider, a man who came to our medical school, to give us a lecture on contraceptive techniques, and the Catholic women were excluded from this lecture, they couldn't attend even if they wanted to. . . . We also had an ob/gyn clinic in med school as part of our clinical training, and we could not write down for the patients the name and address of the Planned Parenthood clinic in town. Nor could we write the name 'Planned Parenthood' on the chalkboard, but we could write the address without the name on the board and point to it and they had to write it down and they could go there. . . . Some of us decided to go down to Planned Parenthood and learn how to fit diaphragms. We went down on our own time."

But coexisting with this legacy of antiabortion attitudes was the reality of an unceasing demand for abortions on the part of women patients. And as the above quotation suggests, physicians in practice in the pre-*Roe* era were typically not in a position to offer patients adequate contraceptive services. Birth control was technically illegal in the United States for much of the twentieth century. Laws prohibiting the dissemination of information and services about contraception were covered under the same antiobscenity statutes – the notorious Comstock laws – that had also criminalized abortion. Though some individual states gradually abolished these laws, and various Supreme Court decisions modified them – for example, allowing physicians to prescribe contraception as a means of preventing disease – it was not until the *Griswold v. Connecticut* decision in 1965 that the "right" of married couples to practice contraception was established (followed in 1972, with the *Eisenstadt v. Baird* decision, which established similar rights of the unmarried).[15]

Birth control before *Griswold*, then, showed a number of similarities to abortion before *Roe*, including a highly complex, often stormy, relationship with organized medicine. A birth control "movement" – whose best known figure was Margaret Sanger – emerged in the United States around World War I which sought to have contraception legalized and birth control services made widely available, to women of all income levels, and irrespective of marital status. Sanger's original vision had been to establish a national fleet of community-based clinics, where women practitioners – mostly nurses – would offer birth control information and services, especially the diaphragm, which began to be available in the United States in the 1920s. The goal was to provide not only contraception, but also information and counseling on sexuality. This vision was impossible to sustain, however, because of the repeated closings of her clinics by the police (on charges of violating the Comstock laws), and ultimately Sanger and her allies were forced to accept physician control of these clinics. Yet the medical profession as a whole was slow to accept the principle of routine use of contraception. It was not until 1937 (more than twenty years after Sanger and other birth control activists had raised the issue) that the AMA officially endorsed contraception as an element of "normal sexual hygiene in married life," while reaffirming the principle that birth control services should remain under strict medical supervision.[16]

In another parallel with the abortion situation, before *Griswold*, many sympathetic physicians (admittedly with far lesser penalties to fear) repeatedly defied the law to make contraceptive services available. For example, at a time when New York state law permitted the prescribing of contraception only for "medical indications," Sanger's flagship New York clinic routinely offered women with no such indications "quiet referrals" to private physicians who would fit diaphragms under these conditions.[17] Countless physicians in private practice across the country similarly violated the law by providing contraception to unmarried women or, simply, "healthy" women. We can conclude therefore that with birth control, as with abortion,

social class was decisive in obtaining services: women with resources, such as an existing relationship with a private physician,
had a better chance of obtaining these forbidden services.

A final intriguing parallel between abortion and birth control provision is the professional stigma that was originally associated with
each. The historical record makes clear that a number of physicians
who early on allied with the birth control movement were ostracized
by their colleagues in ways that prefigured in some respects what
would later happen to physicians who provided abortions. When Dr.
Hannah Stone, for example, accepted the position of medical director
of Sanger's main clinic, she was forced to give up her staff privileges
at a prestigious New York hospital, and for a number of years she was
denied membership in the New York Academy of Medicine.[18]

The combination of the scarcity of birth control, the rise in
premarital sex, and the desire for smaller families that characterized
most of the twentieth century[19] meant that physicians were faced
with a steady stream of women seeking abortions. But as medical
knowledge about the management of pregnancy increased after
World War II, physicians faced the dilemma that pregnancies decreasingly posed clear-cut "threats to the life of the mother" or even
serious jeopardy to her physical health. Hence, a greater proportion
of requests for hospital-approved abortions were on more ambiguous grounds, such as mental health considerations. As Kristin Luker
has pointed out, this development exacerbated strains among two
different groups of physicians – those generally morally opposed to
abortion, who wanted their colleagues to adhere to the most rigid
interpretations of the laws governing approved abortions, and those
who pushed for broader, and more discretionary, policies.[20]

As an attempt to further rationalize the abortion decision – and to
protect themselves in the uncertain legal climate described above –
physicians in the years after World War II developed the "therapeutic
abortion committee" system. These committees, theoretically, would
rise above the more informal – and, arguably, arbitrary – manner in
which decisions to perform hospital-approved abortions had previously been made. While till then, a physician merely needed the approval of two colleagues, abortions would now be granted on the ba-

sis of strict guidelines. Alan Guttmacher, one of the most influential ob/gyns of the era, is credited with innovating this system at Mt. Sinai Hospital in Baltimore in 1945, and it became widely copied across the country.[21]

Under this new system, hospitals formed committees, typically consisting of both ob/gyns and colleagues from other departments, and physicians seeking abortions for their patients would present their cases at a weekly meeting. These therapeutic abortion committees, nearly all commentators agree, did not meet original expectations. In many instances, the committees, fearful of attracting unwanted attention, were extremely cautious, developing informal – if not formal – quota systems for the number of abortions permitted in a given year. Critics of the system moreover charged that the private patients of physicians – as opposed to ward patients – were being disproportionately favored for the abortion slots that did exist. These critics also pointed to the sterilization requirements that frequently accompanied a committee-approved abortion. Not surprisingly, the number of hospital-based abortions went down dramatically after the formation of such committees. Lawrence Lader, a journalist and prominent abortion rights activist in the 1960s, caustically remarked on the estimated drop in hospital-approved abortions from about thirty thousand in 1940 to about eight thousand in 1965, attributing this reduction to "one of the greatest cases of jitters ever to afflict the medical profession."[22]

Yet simultaneous with the "tightening up" of legal abortion provision in some locales was an expansion in others. Hospitals in some regions had highly differing rates of approval through the committee than did others in the same state. Some states, with the approval of physicians, liberalized their abortion statutes to permit abortion in the case of mental health indications; in practice, this often came to mean that anyone with the money to obtain the requisite two consultations with a psychiatrist could obtain an abortion. Hence physicians were able to send those patients who could afford it to other states for abortions, just as they had for some time been making referrals to places outside the United States, such as Puerto Rico, Mexico, Japan, and England.

MEDICAL MOBILIZATION

The cumulative effect of all the events described above was to render meaningless for most physicians – whatever their personal views – the notion that their profession had any coherent policy on abortion. Physicians in practice in the 1950s and 1960s saw the enormously arbitrary workings of the supposedly neutral committee system. They saw their colleagues on the one hand denounce "filthy abortionists," yet at the same time constantly be on the search for reliable providers of illegal abortion to whom to send their patients or family members. They realized that what was considered both "immoral" and "illegal" in one state, e.g., an abortion on mental health grounds, was perfectly acceptable practice in a neighboring state.

And if the medical profession had no coherent view on abortion, "society" as a whole seemed to have even less. While abortion, from the forties through the sixties, was a topic for only covert discussion, carrying associations of secrecy and shame, this certainly did not prevent women – including the middle- and upper-class wives, girlfriends, sisters-in-law, and friends of many male doctors – from seeking them. Every one of the thirty-five male physicians interviewed for this study had been approached by either family members or friends begging for information on how to obtain an abortion. The ten women, because of their presumed higher degree of sympathy, were besieged by requests, and among this group at least four had had an illegal abortion themselves.

Perhaps most untenable of all for physicians was the erratic and unpredictable legal consequences of abortion from the 1940s through 1973. Physicians simply did not *know* when a district attorney, for whatever political reasons, or an antiabortion colleague, as in the case of the San Francisco Nine, would choose to question certain kinds of abortion that had hitherto been officially ignored.

Out of both genuine sympathy for women seeking abortion and professional self-interest, therefore, more and more physicians began to fight to liberalize abortion laws. Physicians sympathetic to abortion reform, including Alan Guttmacher, were instrumental in starting one of the first "pro-choice" organizations, the Association for the Study of Abortion (originally the Association for Humane Abortion) in 1965.[23] Many physicians threw their support behind a model statute for abortion proposed by the prestigious American Law Institute. The ALI model permitted legal abortion on three grounds: if the pregnancy "would gravely impair the physical or mental health of the mother"; if the child was likely to be born with "grave physical or mental defects"; and if the pregnancy resulted from rape or incest.[24]

Other physicians, who found the ALI proposal too constrictive, became involved in the more militant efforts of the period, led by an abortion rights movement (joined, in turn, by a newly reemergent feminist movement), to repeal all existing abortion laws.[25] Starting in 1967, a significant breakthrough in abortion law came about in some states, as Colorado and California significantly liberalized their abortion laws. The outright repeal of abortion law in New York and Washington, D.C. in the early 1970s meant that in the several years before *Roe* there were already examples of widespread abortion provision to a "normal" population, and interested physicians from all over the country observed the events in those places closely. The founding of the first generation of freestanding clinics took place in these immediate pre-*Roe* years, and flagship clinics such as Preterm in Washington, D.C. became both national and international training sites for physicians committed to learning abortion procedures.

Physicians participated in these broader political movements at the same time that considerable abortion-related activity was occurring within the medical profession in the 1950s and 1960s. After years of attempting to distance itself from the abortion issue, Planned Parenthood Federation of America, with which many influential ob/gyns of the era had become affiliated, became increasingly vocal about the need for changes in abortion policy. As a result of this mobilization among abortion-sympathetic physicians, two highly significant conferences on abortion were held in the two decades before *Roe*: one sponsored by Planned Parenthood in New York in 1955, and one sponsored by the Association for the Study of Abortion in Hot Springs, Virginia in 1968. Each of these conferences focused on the medical, legal, ethical, and social aspects of abortion, both in the

United States and elsewhere. Given the animosity that many physicians of this era felt toward the "abortionist," a particularly noteworthy feature of each conference is that the speaker's platform was offered to a noted physician provider of illegal abortions – L. Cottrell Timanus at the Planned Parenthood conference and Robert Spencer at the Hot Springs conference.

Timanus was one of the best-known providers of illegal abortion of the pre-*Roe* era. He was based in the Washington-Baltimore area and was used by many physicians in that region as a referral source in the 1930s and 1940s. He is estimated to have provided some thousands of abortions. At the Planned Parenthood conference, Alan Guttmacher, who had become acquainted with Timanus years earlier while at John Hopkins University, introduced his old acquaintance in the following words: "Our next speaker, Dr. Timanus, has been very gracious in coming here to give us a frank exposition of the work as it was carried on by, in my estimation, an extremely competent abortionist. Dr. Timanus has been known to me for almost three decades, and I value his friendship." Timanus then gave a talk in which he detailed both the socioeconomic characteristics of a group of 5200 women he had aborted, as well as the techniques he used. He reported that in this group there were two deaths – "about 0.04 percent mortality"; the actual cause of death in both cases was never determined.[26]

Robert Spencer openly practiced abortion in Ashland, Pennsylvania, a small coal mining town, from 1923 until his retirement in 1967. His abortion practice, which drew women from all over the East Coast and beyond, was part of a very busy general practice. A number of written accounts of Spencer suggest a particularly admired "family doctor." He, for example, was one of the only local physicians willing to go down into the mine when an accident had occurred. Local Ashland residents, even those opposed to abortion, nonetheless remained his loyal patients. Spencer and his wife were also quite active in community affairs, such as the Rotary Club. This level of integration into the life of a small town may explain why Spencer was never convicted of performing abortion, even though he was several times brought to trial. In his most serious confrontation with the law, he was tried for the death of a patient, a woman who had died – apparently of a heart attack – while he was administering anesthesia prior to the abortion. On this occasion, also, a jury acquitted him. This case was the only death that occurred in the over thirty thousand abortions that Spencer had performed.[27]

Spencer became ill at the time of the Hot Springs conference and was unable to attend, but the published proceedings of the conference contain the paper he had planned to present. Like Timanus, he reported both on the socioeconomic characteristics of patients, including the reasons they offered for wanting an abortion, as well as a detailed account of his methods. Spencer's descriptions of his methods are of particular interest, because he successfully used techniques that proved very risky in the hands of other illegal abortionists. Besides the anesthesia death, Spencer claimed that the only other significant difficulties he encountered in performing thirty thousand abortions were uncontrollable hemorrhage in one patient, who required a hysterotomy, and the necessity to repeat the D. & C. procedure on two patients. A small number of patients – "not more than one in a hundred" – returned to his office after their abortions because of minor complications. He did acknowledge, however, the high likelihood that some patients experienced problems after leaving Ashland. ("In the absence of any reports of serious complications, it is assumed that they were probably mild to moderate.")

Spencer's initial method when he began in the 1920s was to use "Leunbach paste" – an abortifacient paste developed in Europe that became a common method of illegal abortion in the United States. After sulfa drugs became available in the 1930s, Spencer modified his procedure to include a D. & C., while still using some of the paste, on the theory that it made the D. & C. technically easier and less bloody. His practice was to inject the patient with the paste in the evening, perform the D. & C. the following morning, and release her in the midafternoon after a period of rest and observation.

In his paper, Spencer described his careful screening of potential patients – he did not accept anyone more than twelve weeks pregnant, or who had other medical conditions, such as uterine fibroids, that would make a D. & C. risky. He had a personal conference with each patient before her release, at which time he warned her of possible complications, gave postoperative instructions and a packet of medications, and offered birth control advice (late in his practice, after oral contraception became available, he offered each patient a prescription for the pill). He reported that his initial fees had ranged from $5 to $25 and gradually stabilized at $100 during World War II (in an era in which some other providers of illegal abortion were routinely charging upwards of $1000); he added that he had a sliding-scale system and that no one was ever turned away for lack of funds. Finally, he mentioned that because his patients were required to stay overnight in Ashland, due to the timing of his procedure, and because area lodgings were not open to black women (about 2 percent of his patient load) he had expanded his clinic to include overnight accommodations.[28]

That Timanus and Spencer were invited to present papers at two such prestigious medical gatherings is noteworthy in several respects. Most fundamentally, these invitations indicate how eager some mainstream physicians were for the kind of *information* – on techniques of out-of-hospital abortion, on outcomes on a large number of otherwise healthy patients – that only those who had done illegal abortions were in a position to give. Most ob/gyns in the 1950s and 1960s, we must recall, had performed few abortions and typically only on women who were seriously ill. The interest shown at the conferences in such data is further indication that an influential group within American medicine saw the legalization of abortion as not only desirable, but inevitable – and realized that they needed to prepare themselves for this eventuality.

But beyond the intrinsic interest in the experiences of the two illegal abortionists, their appearances at these gatherings carried symbolic weight. The public praise that such a revered figure as Alan Guttmacher gave Timanus, his declaration of their "friendship," and the subsequent publication of Timanus's and Spencer's presentations in two landmark conference volumes would seem to mark a crucial change in the relationship between mainstream physicians and the "abortionist." Or, to put it more precisely, the positive reception accorded Timanus and Spencer publicly acknowledged the willingness of at least one wing within mainstream medicine to make *distinctions* among physician providers of illegal abortion.[29] Rather than decrying them as one vast collection of incompetents and "butchers," as earlier generations of "regular" physicians had done, some within the elite world of obstetrics/gynecology were now saying publicly what some had long acted on privately: there were "good" illegal abortionists as well as "bad" ones. And "good" referred to the medical competence of the abortionist as well as to his ethics. Thus, someone like Robert Spencer, who kept scrupulous medical records, displayed appropriate caution in deciding which cases he could handle, operated in a medical setting in which he could hospitalize patients if necessary and receive help from colleagues, and, above all else, had compiled an extraordinary safety record, was someone who merited medical respect. Beyond that, his sliding-scale policy with respect to fees and his progressive stance toward minority patients undermined the stereotype of the avaricious abortionist, who cared only about money.

The introduction to U.S. physicians of the vacuum suction method of abortion was another significant aspect of the Hot Springs conference. The presentation on the suction machine was given by Franc Novak, an ob/gyn from Yugoslavia. The vacuum suction method, initially developed in the Soviet Union in 1927, had been used and refined in Eastern Europe and China in the subsequent decades. The enthusiasm generated by this method was due to its obvious superiority, in ease and safety, over the D. & C. As Novak said in his presentation, "When the gynecologist who knows only the conventional D. & C. method first sees the apparatus in action, he is impressed by the cleanness, apparent bloodlessness, speed, and simplicity of the operation. While a D. & C. gives the impression of rude artisan's work, an abortion performed with suction gives the impression of a simple mechanical procedure." Novak went on to report the lessened blood loss experienced by the patient, as well as the dramatically lowered risk of perforation of the uterus – the chief risk of the D. & C. He claimed that at his hospital there had been one report of perforation in twelve thousand abortions using suction, compared to a rate of one in five hundred with the D. & C.[30]

The dissemination of this new technique was greatly facilitated in the United States by a small family foundation in Delaware, the Lalor Foundation. The head of the foundation, C. Lalor Burdick, was deeply interested in contraceptive issues and while traveling in Europe had met Novak and watched him perform several operations using the vacuum suction method. Burdick sponsored Novak's trip to the Hot Springs conference and produced a medical training film on the use of the vacuum method, featuring a British physician, Dorothea Kerslake, which he made widely available to hospitals and medical schools in the United States. His foundation also underwrote the cost of the vacuum suction machines for a number of hospitals that were performing abortions in the late 1960s and early 1970s.[31]

A final noteworthy aspect of the Hot Springs meeting was the special session on "Abortion and Womankind," composed of all women panelists, in which the speakers were charged to "approach the [abortion] question as women." The fact of such a panel – a rarity in the medical culture of the 1960s – is an indication of the incipient recognition, on the part of conference organizers, of abortion's special status as an issue of gender inequality. And some of the speakers did use the occasion to speak in strong feminist language: "[Abortion] is a right so fundamental, so personal to women, that its denial nullifies the right to freedom and to security of their person and of their families," said one.[32]

As a consequence of the increasing interest in "population control" issues in the developing world, on the part of both the U.S. government and numerous private organizations in the 1950s and 1960s, the medical community in the United States became further involved in abortion-related activity. One measure of the legitimacy that family planning programs had now achieved – in contrast to their embattled status in earlier years – was that by 1963, two former presidents, Harry Truman and Dwight Eisenhower, agreed to be honorary chairmen of a Planned Parenthood fundraising campaign.[33] While the primary aim of population organizations in that period was to disseminate birth control methods, there were also attempts to make available to Third World health care providers the euphemistically named "menstrual extraction kits" – which provided early abortions.

These kits consisted of a hand-held suction pump and a plastic, and hence far more flexible, cannula (a tube for insertion into the uterus) than the metal ones that had previously been used in abortions. This technology was felt to be particularly suited for the developing world because the hand-held pump was not dependent on electricity. The more flexible cannula, moreover, would dramatically cut down the risk of injury in very early abortions and also make the procedure less painful (and would therefore not require general anesthesia). Furthermore, it was believed that with the proper supervision and training, health care workers below the rank of physician could safely perform such procedures up through eight weeks of pregnancy.[34] And here again, the experience of illegal providers of abortion in the U.S. was utilized. The plastic cannula was developed by Harvey Karman, a well-known figure in abortion provision in the 1960s. Karman was a psychologist from California who himself performed many illegal abortions. Like Spencer and Timanus, Karman had collegial relationships with mainstream medical figures with whom he shared his technological innovations. The Karman cannulas became widely used not only in developing countries, but in the United States as well, as they became adapted to the standard suction machines.[35]

Given the fervent antiabortion stance that would come to characterize official U.S. policies toward international family planning starting in 1980, with the election of Ronald Reagan, it is interesting to recollect the dramatically different atmosphere – and policies – of just a few years earlier. Tania Meadows, one of the physicians interviewed for this study, was at a 1972 meeting in Hawaii, sponsored by AID (Agency for International Development): "It was about abortion technology in the Third World. AID had literally rooms full of these kits! The kits consisted of the 50cc syringe, a variety of cannulas and instructions on how to do abortions. This was an international meeting. People came from the Pacific Basin, from all over Latin America. It's incredible to think of AID spending this kind of money now on that!" In short, at a time when abortion was still officially illegal in the United States, a federal agency was drawing on the experiences of illegal abortionists to spread accessible abortion technology to the developing world.[36] For physicians involved in international family planning circles, such events as this AID meeting in 1972 were further confirmation of the seemingly inevitable move toward legalization of abortion in the United States.

THE *ROE* DECISION AND MEDICAL EQUIVOCATION

By 1970, the AMA, responding to a variety of forces – the growing visibility of both the population control movement and the abortion rights movement, and, most of all, the increasing frustration with illegal abortion voiced by physicians themselves – adopted a resolution endorsing liberalized abortion laws. The language of this resolution made clear the medical profession's discomfort with abortion activists of that period (mostly outside medicine) who were advocating the repeal of all abortion laws, and especially with the feminist wing of the abortion rights movement, with its call for "abortion on demand." The AMA resolution stated that abortion policy should be based on "sound clinical judgment" and "the best interest of the patient," rather than "mere acquiescence to the patient's demand."[37]

Other discussions at the 1970 AMA meeting revealed how difficult the abortion issue was for many within medicine, because of the fusion of the already charged issue of gender politics with that of the equally explosive issue of "demedicalization." In the late 1960s and early 1970s, a number of "radical health movements" were challenging physicians' prerogatives and authority in a variety of areas; prominent among these movements was a women's health movement that was especially critical of conventional medical practices (and often of the male physician himself) in the area of reproductive health.[38] For some physicians, already wary of these efforts, legal abortion had the potential to subvert the traditional relationship of physician and patient, rendering the former into a mere "technician" who would do the patient's bidding. At the 1970 AMA convention – as feminist groups supporting legal abortion picketed outside the convention hall – one doctor complained, "Legal abortion makes the patient truly the physician: she makes the diagnosis and establishes the therapy."[39]

Indeed, this concern about the potential of legal abortion to dramatically change the relationship between doctor and patient was felt even by those physicians who led efforts to promote legal abortion. For example, a public statement by one hundred professors of obstetrics, issued several months before the *Roe* decision was announced, urged the medical community to begin the necessary preparations to meet the profession's "responsibility" to provide abortions, in light of the changing abortion climate. Yet the statement also acknowledged the difficulties that many of their colleagues would experience: "For the first time, except perhaps for cosmetic surgery, doctors will be expected to do an operation simply because the patient asks that it be done."[40] Similarly, Alan Guttmacher, perhaps the single most important medical activist on behalf of legal abortion before *Roe*, voiced his discomfort, at a session of the 1968 ASA conference, at the prospect of abdicating his role as medical advisor and simply acting as a "rubber stamp" for a woman seeking an abortion.[41] At this same session, Robert Hall, another highly influential physician activist of the era, made a prediction that, as we shall see, was eventually to ring true for a number of those interviewed for this study. After stating his belief that the woman seeking an abortion should receive some counseling—but not necessarily from physicians—Hall went on to say, "Then if she still wants the abortion she should have it. When it comes to the doctor, I think he is eventually going to be no more than a technician. This may be humiliating to him. But it is his unavoidable plight if we are to grant women their inherent right to abortion."[42]

Despite its reservations, the AMA's endorsement of liberalized abortion laws did represent a significant shift, given that a century earlier the organization had spearheaded the drive to criminalize abortion. But this official shift, and indeed the legalization of abortion that ocurred shortly thereafter in 1973, did not "resolve" the abortion issue. The *Roe* decision neither brought American women full access to abortion nor did it end the longstanding ambivalence about abortion within medical circles.

One of the most striking features of the period immediately after *Roe* was the failure of the majority of U.S. hospitals to establish abortion services: by 1977, only 31 percent of all non-Catholic hospitals provided any abortion services. Of the total number of abortions performed that year, hospitals accounted for 27 percent, freestanding clinics 69 percent, and the remaining 4 percent were performed in physicians' offices. (By 1994, as mentioned earlier, the percentage of all abortions offered in hospitals had dropped to 7 percent.) In the immediate post-*Roe* period, as now, abortion facilities tended to cluster in urban areas, posing a particular hardship for rural women.[43]

The low number of hospital-based abortions exacerbated another problem of abortion provision which became quickly evident in that era – the lack of routine training in abortion procedure for residents in obstetrics and gynecology. One 1976 study concluded that more than four out of ten residents did not receive such training.[44] In part, this lack of training could be explained, as I will shortly discuss, by resistance on the part of residency directors; additionally, however, such training was impossible to provide if hospitals were not supplying an adequate number of abortion cases.

Just as most hospitals failed to establish abortion services after *Roe*, many private practitioners in that period were reluctant to provide abortions, or did so very selectively. As one sociological observer put it, in discussing a crucial aspect of *Roe*, "a woman's right to choose the procedure is always circumscribed by the physician's right not to perform it."[45] In an important series of papers studying abortion provision in the state of Maryland in 1975, Constance Nathanson and Marshall Becker found individual physicians' attitudes to be a crucial determinant of whether abortions could be obtained in a particular community. The researchers found that religion was the most powerful predictor of whether physicians would provide abortions, but "satisfaction" with one's patients also strongly affected this decision. The more "liberal" physicians (as measured by questions on women's roles and reproductive freedom) were relatively more likely to provide abortions – but to their own private patients. As the authors stated, the abortions were performed as an "accommodation" for "women of their own social status with whom a prior personal or professional relationship exists."[46] Medicaid patients by and large were not accepted by this group. Therefore, the accessibility of abortion continued to vary according to class, as it had before legalization: in the pre-*Roe* era, many of the physicians who were willing to perform illegal abortions typically did them only for women in their own personal or professional networks.

Similarly, Nathanson and Becker found the availability of hospital-based abortions to depend on individual obstetricians' attitudes. In a pattern that was common in other states as well, most of the abortions done in Maryland in 1976 (68 percent) were performed in only six hospitals. Attempting to explain why so few abortions were performed in other hospitals, and why the proportion of hospital abortions in that state declined by 57 percent between 1973 and 1976, the authors concluded that it was the result of the negative attitudes of the physicians affiliated with the hospitals with low abortion rates, rather than the organizations' capacities or resources.[47] Similarly, Robert Hall, commenting on the fact that in New York City shortly after legalization most hospital abortions were done by a small number of doctors, said: "The rest of the staff regards these doctors with esteem not markedly higher than that previously reserved for the back street abortionist."[48]

Just as many individual physicians and hospitals distanced themselves from abortion in the immediate aftermath of *Roe*, influential medical organizations were reticent, to say the least. In a survey taken in 1976 of major national associations in health and related fields, twenty-two out of the thirty-six responding organizations reported taking no actions of the type that would be normally expected after such a major policy change; these groups issued no public statements, guidelines, or standards on abortion after the handing down of *Roe*. These silent groups included the Association of American Medical Colleges, the Joint Commission on Accreditation of Hospitals, the National Board of Medical Examiners, and the American Association for Hospital Planning. The AMA's only major statement on abortion in this period was a resolution adopted by its House of Delegates in June 1973 stipulating that abortions be performed only by licensed physicians in accredited hospitals, and that "physicians with conscientious objections to abortion be free to withdraw from these cases." The only health organizations that took an active part in debate about abortion policy at this time were the American Public

Health Association and the American College of Obstetricians and Gynecologists. The APHA in 1973 issued a *Comprehensive Guide for Abortion Services*, stressing, among other things, the importance of making abortion services "readily available in the community of residence of all patients in need of the service." ACOG, already on record in support of abortion reform before the *Roe* decision, issued an official statement after the decision urging that first trimester abortions be performed either in hospitals or in licensed clinics with hospital back-up services.[49]

In sum, we can conclude that in the immediate aftermath of *Roe* the medical leadership in the United States was not so much "opposed" to abortion as it was, in the words of some observers, "equivocal."[50] Mainstream medicine's response to *Roe* might be characterized as opportunities lost; the 1970s *could* have been a time of massive education about abortion issues at state and local as well as national levels, directed both toward health care institutions and legislators. And though some within medicine in this period did publicly urge their colleagues to take a proactive stance toward abortion provision,[51] for the most part medical leadership remained silent.

In seeking to explain why abortion services and training remained so marginalized from mainstream medicine after the *Roe* decision, Philip Darney, a physician who is a leading student of abortion provision, points to the atypical history of the innovation and dissemination of abortion techniques – and to the enduring stigma within medicine that was associated with the pre-*Roe* "abortionist." As described by Darney, the typical route for the dissemination of a new surgical technique is that it is developed by an academic (who often has received research funds for this purpose), described at medical meetings and in relevant professional literature, and taught by the innovator to colleagues and students, who in turn teach it to their students. This conventional path, of course, was not the case with abortion. Those with the most expertise in abortion technique immediately after *Roe* were not professors of obstetrics and gynecology, but those who had extensive experience performing illegal abortions. And although some within mainstream medical circles were extremely eager to make contact with these individuals – inviting Drs. Spencer and Timanus to present at major medical conferences, for example – for the majority of those who directed ob/gyn residencies, abortionists were to be shunned. As Darney put it, "Academic departments of obstetrics and gynecology [did not] welcome skilled abortionists to their ranks. Even though abortion now was legal, a stigma remained on those who had earlier performed illegal abortions."[52] The lack of experienced teachers in residency programs, plus the evident disapproval of many senior physicians, led to a situation in which those who wished to learn abortion techniques increasingly sought training in the freestanding clinics that were proliferating in this period.

The situation after *Roe*, then, was one in which the medical mainstream's reluctance to become involved in abortion led to an increasing dependence on the freestanding clinic as the major site for both abortion services and training. Though the freestanding clinic in many ways has been a very positive model of abortion services, I will argue that this heavy reliance on clinics has further isolated abortion from dominant medical institutions – a development with negative consequences. In the immediate post-*Roe* era, as in the present, that majority of ob/gyns who count themselves "pro-choice" but who do not provide abortions can rationalize their behavior by assumimg that "the clinics" will take care of the abortion problem.

Another development of the years following *Roe* which doubtless had a chilling effect on some physicians' willingness to become engaged with abortion was the emergence of an antiabortion movement as a significant force in American politics. During the presidential administration of Jimmy Carter, the issue of federal funding of abortions for Medicaid recipients became highly controversial, eventually culminating in a Supreme Court decision striking down such policies.[53] During the years of the presidencies of Ronald Reagan and George Bush (from 1980 to 1992), official attempts to restrict legal abortion became far more widespread, with both presidents on record as favoring an overturning of the *Roe* decision. During the Reagan-Bush years, moreover, abortion became one of the most visible, and divisive, issues in domestic politics, as the two presidents – in response to their backing from right-wing conservatives – put in place a number of policies, ranging from the abortion "litmus tests" applied to virtually all high-level political appointees and judicial nominees, to the notorious "gag rule," which stipulated that family planning clinics receiving federal funding could not counsel patients about abortion.[54] Though it was not until the late 1980s that the most violent wing of the antiabortion movement became a significant factor in abortion politics, it did become clear to medical professionals quite quickly after *Roe* that the decision would bring ample political controversy. And the medical community in the United States, it can safely be said, was (and is) a largely conservative one, not fond of such controversy.

This review of the relationship of U.S. medicine and abortion in the nineteenth and twentieth centuries thus reveals a profession deeply ambivalent about abortion. Abortion practices in the pre-*Roe* period created a complex legacy for physicians active after *Roe*, given the enduring images of inept "quacks" and "butchers" and the associations with criminality and greed. Moreover, the seeming inseparability of abortion from radical social movements – the feminist movement at one pole, antiabortionists at the other – was a further incentive for many physicians to avoid performing abortions. Furthermore, as I have shown, even sympathetic physicians were troubled by the prospect of abortion becoming a routine procedure for healthy women and thus requiring little skill. Yet weighed against these negative features was the reality that most physicians – ob/gyns and family practitioners in particular – saw in their practices in the decades before *Roe*: an unending stream of women, including those in the physicians' own personal lives, who wanted abortions and would often go to extremely dangerous lengths to get them. Hence the quite odd split that characterized U.S. medicine in the period immediately surrounding *Roe* (and still does today): a majority of physicians voiced support of abortion as a valid choice for a woman to make yet were far less supportive of those who provided these abortions.

Against this backdrop of a divided and ambivalent medical profession, the next few chapters of this book relate the experiences of a group of abortion-sympathetic physicians ("physicians of conscience," as I have called them) whose careers spanned the pre- and post-*Roe* eras.

CHAPTER THREE

"The Lengths to Which Women Would Go": Encountering Abortion Before *Roe*

Physicians embarking on medical careers between 1940 and 1970, including those interviewed for this book, were coming into a profession increasingly torn about abortion. The longstanding negative feelings about the "abortionist" within medical circles coexisted with a growing conviction among at least some influential segments of the profession, who began calling for abortion reform and preparing themselves for eventual legalization, that the status quo on abortion was unworkable and unreasonable. Young physicians in practice or training in the pre-*Roe* era thus faced difficult – at times, untenable – conflicting pressures. On the one hand, it was very clear that to become involved in illegal abortion was, at worst, to jeopardize a medical career and risk imprisonment, and, short of that, to become identified with an activity that was historically despised by many of one's colleagues. On the other hand, *not* to engage in abortion in some fashion came to feel like complicity in a system that, as one subject put it, "was full of death and injury – all of it so utterly unnecessary." Such direct encounters with the realities of illegal abortion – in their personal lives, as well as professional ones – were central in securing the commitment of this group to abortion provision.

A number of the men interviewed for this study experienced the unwanted pregnancy of their wives or girlfriends and the resultant frantic search for an abortion. Four of the women interviewed themselves underwent illegal abortions. Tania Meadows was several years out of college, in a "difficult marriage," working on the West

Coast and planning for medical school when she became pregnant in 1953. "I started this search for an illegal abortionist which took me from the West Coast to New York. I interviewed a lot of people and saw a lot of undesirable situations. . . . Ultimately I found a very good ob/gyn on Lexington Ave, who for $500 took me in after hours and did a D. & C. . . . It was a very powerful experience in my life. I think I was making up my mind that this is something I might want to work on someday." In a note that Meadows sent to me shortly after our interview, she elaborated on this experience, saying, "One persistent thought I had while performing abortions throughout my career was that I was paying back the universe in some way for my luck in finding a competent doctor abortionist for myself, when I was twenty-three years old, which enabled me to go to medical school. It felt very lifesaving at the time."

Ethel Bloom's experience with illegal abortion was more unpleasant than Meadows's, though it had the similar effect of making her highly sympathetic to her patients' needs when she later started medical practice. Bloom was nineteen in 1943, recently married and about to start medical school when she found out she was pregnant. "I asked this doctor I knew, a wonderful progressive doctor, but there was nothing he would do. I had a friend, Rachel, whose mother was a nurse in New York, and we got an address from the gynecologist the mother worked with. Rachel came with me. I remember this toothless woman coming to the door, she was supposed to be the nurse, I remember her putting a cone of ether over my face, and I remember feeling the pain of the abortion. It was the most painful feeling of my life. I remember waking up in this dirty anteroom, and then going back to my friend's apartment. It was a *horrible* experience."

Irving Goodman recalled the situation he and his future wife faced, when both were teenagers in the mid-1940s.

> I was eighteen, she was sixteen. We went to this doctor. . . . I remember he took an instrument out of the closet, it was not sterile. And he started to dilate the cervix, and it was really uncomfortable for her. And he said, "We'll see what happens over the next couple of days." Over the next few days, she became quite ill and infected, a septic situation. . . . We finally ended up telling her own doctor about it who said, "Why didn't you tell

me first, I could have helped you." He sent her to a surgeon, because she
had peritonitis. The surgeon took out her appendix, did a very large incision on her abdomen – almost as if it were punitive – and I heard him
say, "Well, I understand the pregnancy isn't wanted, so I squeezed the
uterus real strongly." And she aborted in the bed the next day.

Goodman, who had given me several reasons during the course of
our interview as to why he was led to abortion work, paused and said,
"This story is the real emotional reason why I said to myself, 'I'm not
going to let this happen to anyone else.'"

Victor Black was in the second year of his ob/gyn residency on the
West Coast in 1963 and thought that the patients he encountered who
had sought illegal abortions "were doing something very wrong. . . .
I remember one patient told me that she had an illegal abortion and I
actually reported her because you were supposed to at that time."
Then he faced a crisis in his own family.

One night I was on call and got a phone call from my wife. She was hys-
terical. I said, "What's wrong with you?" She said, "I think I'm pregnant
again." We had three children. She said, "I'm not going to do this again. I
absolutely refuse to do this again." . . . I said, "What are we going to do?"
She said, "I've got to have an abortion." I said, "I don't know where you
are going to get one, they're illegal." But of course I knew that any one of
my colleagues was capable of doing it. But it was still illegal. After thinking about it for a long time, I decided to do it myself. I didn't want anyone
else to know it was going to be done.

I got the equipment I needed. . . . I borrowed – stole – it from the clinic.
She wasn't very far along, she had just missed her period by a few weeks.
I borrowed a speculum, curette, and syringe and the things that I needed,
and I did it at home. Not under the best of conditions – poor lighting, no
table, no nothing. At first it didn't work. It didn't appear that anything had
happened. I really didn't know what I was doing. I had never done one. It
was the first one I had ever done. I had done D. & C.'s, but I didn't know
what to expect from an abortion. . . . Finally, the procedure did work. She
did abort. She did develop a mild infection and I had to treat her for that,
but fortunately, it all passed. There were no complications. I treated her
with antibiotics. No one else found out about it. It was not necessary to
take her to the hospital or to have anyone else find out about it.

Reginald Berry, an African-American, was a resident in a large general hospital on the East Coast in the late 1960s. Though his hospital, which served a largely minority low-income population, had no shortage of tragedies associated with illegal abortion, for Berry, the most shattering incident of all was the death of one of his fellow residents from an abortion. The woman, whose abortion may have been self-administered, did not admit herself to the hospital until it was too late to save her. Berry and others in his group of residents were grief-stricken, not only because of the loss of a treasured colleague, but because of their conviction that they could have prevented her death had she only turned to them for an abortion. "She was a smart girl, one of the most brilliant girls I have ever known in my life.... She could have had any one of us to do it for her.... I would have done it."

But whether or not they experienced unwanted pregnancies in their own lives, all of the physicians interviewed for this study in the course of their medical training came face to face with the consequences of illegal abortion. For most, the first encounter with illegal abortion came during residency, in the hospital emergency room. Some encountered patients who claimed to be miscarrying–also known medically as "spontaneously aborting"–and the residents' role would be to complete the procedure with a D. & C. As the residents soon came to realize, however, many of these "miscarriages" in fact were abortions that had been initiated outside the hospital. In a minority of cases, moreover, patients would not have an abortion in process–spontaneous or otherwise–and would attempt to simulate such a condition to obtain a D. & C.[1] Alice Wilkins, while a resident in a county hospital in southern California in the 1940s, experienced such a case. "A patient was brought in to the hospital, just streaming with blood. So I went in to complete the procedure, and I became very suspicious when I saw no blood in the vagina at all. It later turned out that her boyfriend worked in a slaughterhouse and had brought home a lot of animal blood to make it appear she was hemorrhaging." Especially when they occurred at the beginning of the young physicians' residencies, such incidents introduced the often naive young doctors to the desperate lengths to which women with unwanted pregnancies were willing to go.

But most patients who appeared at the hospital were in the process of genuine miscarriage, and residents became aware of the wide – often, to them, astonishing – range of methods then in use to induce abortion. Peters McPherson had been a resident at a large public hospital in New Orleans in the 1940s. "We had a woman who somehow or other managed to get a catheter [a hollow tube] into her cervix and poured turpentine down there and literally cooked the lining of her uterus. . . . It was like she got gasoline in there and lit it. We had to take her uterus out." Another common practice for women attempting abortions themselves was to use potassium permanganate tablets. These tablets, widely available over the counter, were placed by pregnant women directly in their vaginas to induce bleeding, and thus to convince medical authorities that they were miscarrying. But as Stan Oliver, who cared for a number of women who had used this method, recalled, "These tablets just eroded the vagina and the women hemorrhaged like hell; [the tablets] lacerated their cervixes." Other doctors reported seeing women in emergency rooms who had used not only the proverbial coat hanger, but also Lysol, broken Coke bottles, catheters, and a variety of other objects.[2] Horace Freeman, who had been a resident in Harlem in the mid-1940s, said, with a sigh, "I have taken everything out of the human vagina that one could imagine ever fitting in there."

Whether their attempted abortions were self-induced or performed by others, many of the abortion patients in emergency rooms were in serious, often life-threatening medical condition because of these attempts. Ken Gordon had been the chief obstetrical resident in the mid-1950s at a public hospital in a large East Coast city. One of Gordon's most powerful memories is of a twenty-two-year-old woman who came to the hospital in septic shock.

What happens there, the infection is so overwhelming, the bacteria produce toxins that lead to a collapse of the cardiovascular system. These patients have no blood pressure, no pulse – in some cases, there is absolutely nothing you can do to reverse the situation. We gave the girl blood, cortisone, hydrocortisone – nothing was working, she was not responsive. We finally figured the only chance we had was to do a hysterectomy. We took her to the O.R., but Anesthesia said, "We won't

give her anesthesia, without getting blood pressure or a pulse. We can't
monitor where we are, and so we might kill her with the anesthesia." So
I had to do something I don't recommend to anybody, which is a hysterectomy under local anesthesia. We got the uterus out – I still have a picture of it in my teaching files – it was basically a bag of pus. We found
a coiled up catheter in there. When we were all done, I was walking
along beside her in the corridor – they were taking her back to her bed.
And one of the tragedies of this septic shock is that people remain lu-
cid until the end, and she was holding my hand, and saying, "Doctor,
help me, I'm dying." And I knew she was, and I knew there was not
a blessed other thing we could do for her, and before she got to her
bed, around midnight, she died, and I have been haunted by that
girl ever since.

For those recipients of illegal abortions who were aborted by the
D. & C. method, perforation of the uterus was a particular hazard.
Describing that procedure, Gordon said, "I always used to tell medical students it was like being blindfolded and trying to scrape wet
cotton balls out of a wet paper bag, and getting all the balls without
tearing the bag.... The uterus was so soft, it was very easy to poke
something through the uterus." Numerous respondents gave horri-
fied accounts – in some cases nearly fifty years after the fact – of the
gruesome aftereffects of botched D. & C.'s. Taylor Buckley, who was
chief resident on an obstetrical ward in a big city general hospital in
the early 1940s, recalled one such case.

A doctor brought her in. He called me and said, "Will you admit her on
your service? She's got a strangulated hernia." I said, "Well, why don't
you send her to general surgery?" He said, "I think it's in your field." She
came in and she had a loop of bowel hanging out of her vagina wrapped
in newspaper and that was the "strangulated hernia." And what he [the
abortionist] did was perforate the uterus. He pulled out the bowel with
his aborting instruments and he thought it was fetal bowel. She had literally over thirty inches of bowel hanging out of her vagina. And the poor
woman should have died from several causes – bowel obstruction, septicemia, and everything else. I operated and did a bowel resection, pulled
this damn dirty bowel out of the uterus and vagina, and she lived. But
many others died.

Residents also saw women who had been aborted using "Leunbach paste," the method that had been used for many years by Robert Spencer, as described in the last chapter. Though Spencer and others[3] apparently used this method quite successfully, in the hands of unskilled practitioners it proved very dangerous. Eugene Fox, while a resident in an Army hospital in the Southwest during World War II, saw a number of women who had crossed the border into Mexico to get the paste. "When the paste got into the bloodstream, it caused immediate hemolysis. The patient just died because all her blood cells broke down. We had several deaths related to that."

A number of respondents in recollecting the consequences of failed abortion attempts they had witnessed pointed out the special intensity that often characterized the relationship between resident and patient in these situations. As Irving Goodman put it, "We were the ones that always had to take care of these patients. . . . We got to be fairly close to the patient because, when you are in your residency, you were really involved with her on a very frequent basis because you had to see her, literally, every two hours. The medical problems were so intense and prolonged that you got to know your patient. And you began to realize the desperation behind which the action was taken."

A corollary to the enormous compassion that many of these young doctors came to feel toward their patients was their enormous rage at the illegal abortionists who had done such inept work. In the case of the massive perforation cited above, for example, the abortionist was known to Taylor Buckley. "He was a referring doctor to our clinic, a general practitioner in our neighborhood. I can still see the bastard's dirty fingernails." Buckley went on to declaim against the "shady, incompetent" abortionists who preyed on vulnerable women, arguing, as many other respondents in this study did, that many were physicians who were simply too inept to succeed at a mainstream medical practice. To be sure, the anger this group felt toward illegal abortionists is complex; as I will discuss in chapter 5, many of these physicians themselves, including Buckley, sought providers of illegal abortion to whom they could refer patients. The challenge, obviously, was to find providers who were both medically competent and ethical.

For many respondents, their increasing recognition of the immense pressures illegal abortions were putting on already burdened hospitals further illustrated the irrationality of abortion restrictions. Numerous subjects recalled the "septic tanks," as residents referred to the special wards in big city hospitals that were reserved for those suffering septicemia (infection of the bloodstream) from illegal abortions. Louise Thomas, a resident in a New York City hospital in the late 1960s, spoke of the "Monday morning abortion lineup": "What would happen is that the women would get their paychecks on Friday, Friday night they would go to their abortionist and spend their money on the abortion. Saturday they would start being sick and they would drift in on Sunday or Sunday evening, either hemorrhaging or septic, and they would be lined up outside the operating room to be cleaned out Monday morning. There was a lineup of women on stretchers outside the operating room, so you knew if you were an intern or resident, when you came in on Monday morning, that was the first thing you were going to do."

The most evocative description of the immense demands placed on public hospitals by illegal abortion came from Renee Giardino, who also had been a resident during the same period in a county hospital in the New York area.

> There were two gyn wards. They were supposed to have thirty-two beds each, but they had to have beds all up and down the hallways. They were always full [because of illegal abortions]. They must have had one hundred and forty beds in those wards. . . . The residents would get duties of twenty-four-hour periods, and in that period, you'd get ten to twelve admissions. They walked into the emergency room bleeding. The first thing the doctor down there did was send them for an X-ray to see what was in their belly – to see if there were knitting needles, hooks, catheters up their belly. . . . Then when they got to the ward, the first thing you did besides examine them was to do a culture for gas gangrene. It was a standard we had, whether they had a fever or not, to take this culture, because if they had gas gangrene, you really had to take drastic measures, like surgery, heavy duty antibiotics, and all that kind of stuff. Until the suction curettage came through, the routine was that you accumulated all the women until two o'clock in the morning when all the

major surgery was done, and the last gunshot wound had been cleared out of the emergency room – then the first-year residents dragged the patients down to the operating room and started doing the D. & C.'s at two o'clock in the morning. That's when the operating room was quiet. . . . There would be two or three operating rooms going at the same time. Between 2:00 and 6:00 A.M. you could get a certain number of D. & C.'s done and clean up the women who weren't septic, scrape their uteruses and get them back upstairs so they could be discharged in a day or two. If they were hemorrhaging profusely, we didn't make them wait until 2:00 A.M. Were they treated badly? I don't know. Everybody at County got treated badly just because we were all so overworked, under stress, and overwhelmed. I don't think they were treated any more badly.

For many of the physicians active in the pre-*Roe* period, the presence of the police in hospital wards was yet another contributing factor to their growing sympathy for abortion patients. The amount of police interrogation of illegal abortion recipients varied widely. Thus, depending on where they were, and when, a number of respondents were routinely forced to deal with police themselves, or to see their patients subjected to cross-examination. Miriam Harkin recalls with remorse her collusion with police in the Midwest in the 1940s. "Well, when I was an intern we'd see these women coming in with illegal abortions. And what bothers me now is that at that stage of my career we were all so indoctrinated how terrible abortion is. If someone came in with an illegal, we would grill her, 'Who did it? Who did it?' We were treating her like a criminal, instead of treating her like a patient. And I participated in that too, and then I thought, 'Am I crazy?! What's going on here?!' "

Some residents learned to circumvent the police whenever feasible because of the strain this imposed on their patients. In New York state in the 1950s and 1960s, for example, physicians in hospitals were required to report "all illegal abortions or suspected illegal ones" to the district attorney. Like many others interviewed, Rosalind Greene, then a resident in a New York hospital, found this requirement untenable. "Women would never admit to having an induced abortion. But that was the law; you were supposed to inform them of anyone you suspected of having an induced abortion. When we saw how they hassled the women, we never called them unless we thought the woman was going to die. If we thought the woman was going to die we knew there would be an investigation afterwards, and therefore we felt we had to call."

For some residents, the experience of seeing a very sick woman refuse to give in to pressure to reveal the name of her abortionist was a transforming experience. Ed Lever, a resident at University Hospital in the Midwest in 1960, recalled such a case, in which he was essentially ordered by his superiors to find out the name of the abortionist in question so a police report could be made.

> This was a young woman with an acute septic abortion, and she had been to a criminal abortionist in Chicago. . . . She was in the process of dying of sepsis and I asked her if she would tell me who did this, and she said no, and she died. And that was the thing that sort of solidified it for me [commitment to legal abortion]. . . . It was starting to impress me that women felt that strongly about an unwanted pregnancy, that they would go to that length, knowing the risks involved – these people must have been awfully frightened and they must have felt very strongly about what they wanted to do. . . . I had always been taught in medical school that physicians were always to be the advocates of the patient and all of a sudden I was no longer an advocate, I was an adversary. That got me terribly upset.

To be sure, some physicians were torn between compassion for abortion patients who were being grilled by policemen and their own rage at incompetent abortionists whose victims would routinely show up in the hospital emergency room. Taylor Buckley, for example, recounted a case in which he thought notifying the police to be highly appropriate. "One case, I recall, where an abortionist infected a girl badly and he pulled an arm off of a fetus that was about twenty weeks, I guess. And she finally came to us with the most horrible story. She had been locked up in his office for forty-eight hours while he was trying to abort her. And he was guzzling bottles of whiskey while taking care of her. And she was in sad shape when she came in. . . . And she very definitely located the guy, he was not far away from the hospital. The cops went and brought him in, and in her feeble state she said, 'That's the man.' All of us had to go to court on that one. But she died and the guy was set free."

Dealing with senior physicians, and particularly with the hospital therapeutic abortion committees, was often another formative experience for the residents. In these hospital situations – working with senior colleagues who were in a position to affect the younger physicians' careers – some of these future abortion providers experienced firsthand the cruelty and hypocrisy that could characterize the medical establishment's response to abortion. Ed Lever had a particularly shattering encounter with his department head.

> A young woman in her twenties, the mother of one child, and a severe diabetic, was admitted to the hospital and I was asked to see her in consultation. . . . She was critically ill, dying in fact from the complications of diabetes. She also was pregnant. I went to the head of my department, Dr. Morgan [not his real name]. . . . I presented the case to him and I said that I thought in order to prolong her life we better terminate the pregnancy and he said, "We don't do that." I said, "What do you mean? We would be doing it to save her life, and there are such statutes on the book," and I went to the library and got the statute and showed it to him, and he said, "We don't do abortions," and she died. And this so upset me. She was going to die eventually but her life could have been prolonged.

Tania Meadows also recalled the callousness of the abortion committee in her West Coast hospital in the early 1960s. "Well, there was a woman who wanted an abortion who was very emotionally disturbed. She was married with one child who had some very severe congenital malformation that was not considered hereditary. They were both on welfare, she and her husband. They were utterly down and out. They were desperate and she was applying for an abortion and was turned down. She was turned down because she was married, and it was felt – I can't remember the exact words the committee used – that a married woman should have her children, and since they had one, another one would 'complete their family.'" The unfairness that Meadows confronted in this abortion committee was profoundly upsetting to her, and, as she later realized, was instrumental in leading her to a "feminist" analysis of the abortion issue. "It was the first time I had really come up against discrimination of the kind that was incomprehensible to me. . . . The people on these committees were really at that time and at that place viewing women as reproductive machines."

The hospital abortion committees often operated on a quota basis, and the residents and young practitioners came to realize that their clinic patients were competing for precious slots with the private patients of their superiors. Virtually everyone interviewed for this study commented on the inherent unfairness of abortion provision before legalization. Thomas Darrow's observation about the small Southern hospital in which he was a resident in the 1960s was typical. "It all depended on who you were. As long as you were the banker's daughter, the doctor's daughter, the golf buddy's daughter, it was always taken care of." Morris Fischer recounts the experience, common to many of those interviewed, of being approached by an antiabortion colleague whose daughter needed an abortion. "I said to him, 'I'll do the abortion and now your daughter will be fresh as a daisy, clean as a pin, and you are relieved of a terrible tragedy that otherwise would have occurred in your family. How do you reconcile that with what you do in the Committee meetings, where you forbid abortions for other patients?' He answered, 'I have a different code for my family.'"[4] Yet another hypocritical twist came with some residents' realization that some of the illegal abortions (presented as miscarriages) that they were called upon to complete had been induced by the attending physicians who were their supervisors – attendings who had, in many cases, shown little sympathy for the clinic patients admitted with incomplete abortions. Horace Freeman recalled that a certain portion of his abortion cases during his residency were "abortions that were started around the corner in the offices of my own attending. . . . It was just a service to the patient, plus a fee."[5]

In contrast, however, to supervisors who were antagonistic to or, at the least, inconsistent about abortion, some of the physicians interviewed for this book had mentors who supported legal abortion, and their beliefs had a lasting impact on their students. Eugene Fox, like the five others in this study who studied under Alan Guttmacher, received a quite different message about abortion than many of the others interviewed. "He discussed this problem in our lectures. . . . He felt abortion was a right women should have. . . . The only birth control we had at that time were the barrier methods. . . . The issue of abortion came up because there were a lot of unplanned pregnancies related to the use of these barrier methods." Louise Thomas, while a medical student in New England in the 1960s, spoke of her "consciousness raising" by professors who were attempting to liberalize abortion laws. "One of my professors – the only woman role model I had in medicine – used to take us students to the legislative hearings on the subjects of abortion and contraception at the state capitol."

For a significant minority (about one third) of those interviewed, their professional experiences in the developing world at an early stage in their careers influenced their decision to become involved in abortion, domestically as well as internationally. Renee Giardino and Simon Ross are representative of those who were profoundly affected by their international work. Giardino went to medical school and completed an internship in the mid-1960s, and in neither stage of her training was abortion a particularly salient issue. She then accepted a two-year fellowship to India, with the intention of returning afterwards to be a general practitioner in a small town. Her assignment in India was to work at a tuberculosis hospital run by the Catholic Church; to her surprise, the nuns constantly urged her to undertake family planning work. "They'd tell me to go talk to that family, tell them how to stop having so many children; they couldn't afford them, couldn't feed them."

After India, Giardino did follow through with her plan to establish a general practice in Ohio. But her experience in India had definitively changed her life course. "I just got really crazy about the population problems in India. . . . I was *so* wiped out by what population was doing to that country. . . . I spent a year doing general practice in Ohio. It was nice – in some ways the most gratifying medical experience I have had – I mean people actually got better! In India they got better for three days and then they got sick again. So Ohio was just marvelous – except this India thing kept flashing back to me, like I just can't be here in this fancy town, making nice money, living in a nice house."

After one year in Ohio, Giardino was hired by a private family planning organization and, after some training, sent to Pakistan to work on a project involving some of the earliest trials of IUDs (intra-uterine devices) in Southeast Asia. The class of IUDs with which she was working were not entirely effective and soon Giardino felt obli-gated to help find illegal abortions for women whom the IUDs had failed. "We were telling them we were going to give them protection from pregnancy and it wasn't working. . . . So we helped them find abortions."

The illegal abortionist whom Giardino found was a very compe-tent one. "Our medical colleagues in Karachi recommended her, that's where they'd send their girlfriends, wives, sisters, whatever. . . . She actually had her office right across from the international air-port. People would fly in, walk across the street, get their abortion, and get back on the next plane, and go home. . . . It was an amazing experience and she was a very good person, and a good doctor. It was my first experience with an illegal abortionist and it was a positive one. She did an excellent job and she knew what she was doing."

Deeply moved by this experience, and by her experience in India, Giardino decided, "I had to be more than a g.p." and returned to the States, where she entered an ob/gyn residency in the New York area.

Simon Ross came from a highly religious and socially conserva-tive background. His feelings about abortion also were deeply influ-enced, at an early point in his career, by his exposure to different cul-tures, as Giardino's had been. In the late 1950s he was working for the U.S. Public Health Service on an Indian reservation in the Southwest.

> I started to get impressed about the problem [family planning] because I
> had a patient – she was blind and had nine children. She would walk in
> several miles for her prenatal care. And I saw her walking one day with
> her white stick along the highway. The rule of law (for employees) on
> the Indian reservation was that you should not pick up any of the Indi-
> ans with your personal car and bring them into the hospital. That was
> my start of ignoring the law, I think. I picked her up and gave her a ride
> into the hospital. And when I talked to her, she said she wanted to be ster-

ilized after she had this baby. She had the last three or four by Caesarean section. And I said, "I think that can be arranged." The time came for the delivery.... The surgeon was Catholic. I said, "This woman has nine children, she's blind, and she certainly shouldn't have any more." He said, "Well, there's no law against having children" and wouldn't do it.

We proceeded to do the Caesarean, and she had titanium mesh all through her abdomen.... I had to use a metal cutter during the operation to get into her abdomen. And then the surgeon did the incision in the uterus and removed the baby.... While he was taking care of the baby, I quickly took care of her tubes, and he never knew it. There was no written permission. I, again, disobeyed the law, so to speak, for her welfare, I felt. She was very, very grateful. That started my interest in family planning and the problem of having too many children.

Ross's experience with Native Americans was followed, in 1957, by several years' work in Korea, at an orphanage near Seoul. Ross claims he was initially hired because of the mystifyingly high death rate of the infants who were brought to the orphanage. "I lost two hundred fifty babies out of five hundred. I started doing autopsies on them; I lost them to pneumocystic occurring pneumonia – the same thing that now kills AIDS patients." Ross began to visit other orphanages around Korea and saw similar high death rates of infants. "I went and walked down rows and rows of these babies. About every fourth one was dying. I talked to people who worked there, and they said, 'They all die.'"

Ross's subsequent investigations suggested to him that these children at the orphanage were not, as he had initially thought, mixed race children of American GIs and Korean women, but rather children of Korean couples who simply could not afford to raise them. According to his informants, fathers would take the several-month-old infants (usually girls) from the mother's side during the night and bring them to police stations, and the police in turn would bring them to the orphanages.

During his stay in Korea, Ross had a very significant encounter with Margaret Roots, a well-known advocate of birth control and a former colleague of Margaret Sanger's.[6] Roots first introduced him to the IUD, which he then made available to Korean patients. On one occasion, she accompanied him to the orphanage in which he was working. "As we walked those aisles, watching babies die – probably out of two hundred babies, twenty were dying right then, from diarrhea – she looked up at me and said, 'It would be better if they had never been born.' I had to stop a minute – it suddenly struck me. I said, 'You're right, even abortion would be better than this.' ... I decided then – this was 1960 – that I was going to do research and work, not only with the IUD, but something in the area of abortion. The IUD was not that effective then. You got women [using the IUD] who got pregnant then."

Ross returned to the United States in the early 1960s and subsequently began providing abortions, which he continued to do after *Roe*. He attributed his decision specifically to his stay in Korea. "I had been so thoroughly convinced, from my Korean experience, that the control of fertility is essential. It's a plain matter of common sense that birth control methods are not that reliable. That they don't take care of every problem in this area. I had seen so many disasters overseas that I thought, American women were not that different from Korean women in the same situation."

Although only some of these physicians had practiced in the developing world, all of them were exposed in the course of their training to extreme poverty in the United States. For the often naive young doctors, most of whom came from the comfortable backgrounds typical of most physicians in the United States, such exposure awakened their sympathy and persuaded them of the necessity of improved birth control and legal abortion. Caleb Barrington, one of eight children from a quite wealthy background, grew up on a large country estate. He recalled the quite different circumstances of those he cared for while a resident in New York City in the 1960s: "It was quite a shock to me to go through the triumph of delivering babies and handing them back to mothers who clearly did not care about these babies and did not want them from the start. People who, when handed their babies, would turn their face to the wall where they already had four or five children, in a single room apartment in New York, in the middle of squalor, and they could not give the kind of care essential for a child to thrive."

Similarly, Howard Wellstone, who had also been a resident in New York, but thirty years earlier, attributed his emerging feelings about abortion to the grinding poverty of his patients. "I was a resident at City Hospital in 1935 in the depths of the Depression. I'd go out [on housecalls after deliveries] and see the women not able to get out of bed for the fourth or fifth day from weakness because of lack of food – in New York! in the United States! I think that was when I became aware that pregnancy for all women was not a joyful or a happy thing. That maybe they should be offered an alternative to pregnancy. Until then, I hadn't really thought about abortion."

Quite obviously, there are many factors that led this group of forty-five physicians to commit to some degree of abortion activity before abortion was legalized, and to remain committed after *Roe*. Some spoke quite movingly of early childhood memories of a beloved relative or family friend dying of an illegal abortion; others, as I have recounted, spoke of their own traumatic searches for a safe abortion. Some attributed their abortion involvement to longstanding family traditions of participation in progressive social movements. Some, as mentioned, had life-changing experiences in the developing world. Some respondents – especially, though not exclusively, female – either explicitly or implicitly used the language of feminism to explain their initial pull toward abortion work.

But none of these factors alone – whether an unwanted pregnancy in their own lives or an identification with progressive social causes – accounts for these physicians' eventual commitment to abortion work. The one experience all these physicians did share, however, was having faced the medical results of illegal abortion. Eugene Fox, describing his reaction to a patient's death early in his residency, captured the defining experience of all these "conscience" physicians: "I could not understand why she died. There were a lot of things I did not know at the time. One of the things I didn't know was the lengths to which some women would go to get an abortion."

CHAPTER FOUR

"I Was Doing It for Reasons of Conscience": Providing Illegal Abortions

Fifteen of the physicians interviewed for this study acknowledge having performed illegal abortions. Because of the ambiguous legal status of abortion in the immediate pre-*Roe* period, it is necessary to clarify what is meant here by "illegal" abortion. I am referring to abortions, whether hospital-based on not, that took place secretly, without any official authorization from medical colleagues. (Others in this study, as I shall discuss in the next chapter, took part in the "gray area" abortions that were sanctioned by hospital therapeutic abortion committees but that nonetheless were done in an uncertain legal environment.) The accounts in this chapter demonstrate both the decency and courage of a group of physicians who operated simultaneously with the better-known "butchers" of the pre-*Roe* era and the enormous constraints upon those who sought to perform illegal abortions responsibly. Apart from the obvious fears of detection, this group faced a situation in which to do some abortions invariably meant being flooded with requests from other desperate women – requests that could inundate a physician's medical practice. Furthermore, the decision to provide illegal abortions meant performing risky, often unfamiliar medical procedures when, by definition, the doctors could not consult with colleagues or easily hospitalize their patients. Their participation in these illegal activities, therefore, made these conscience physicians acutely aware of how ineffectual a response their efforts were to the larger problem of unwanted pregnancies. In short, providing illegal abortions made it even more apparent to this group that it was imperative abortion be legalized.

It is beyond the scope of this book to explain precisely why some, and not others, took this risky step of providing illegal abortions. It is far easier to explain why the majority in this group did *not* provide abortions. By performing abortions before *Roe v. Wade*, physicians were putting their medical careers in jeopardy. They were also risking jail sentences. A number of those interviewed spoke quite persuasively of their reluctance to perform illegal abortions, in spite of the enormous sympathy they felt toward their patients. Miriam Harkin and Alice Wilkins, for example, both were single mothers raising young children and simply felt unable to jeopardize their livelihoods by breaking the law. Ken Gordon, who throughout his career has been an eloquent spokesman for the necessity of legal abortion, articulated a concern echoed by many others interviewed – the fear of being overwhelmed by an unending stream of abortion seekers. As Gordon put it, "I knew if I did one, the floodgates would open."

Before turning to the stories of five physicians who performed illegal abortions on a regular basis, over a period of time, I will describe some of the more sporadic strategies used by those who did not usually accede to requests but who, periodically, could not bear to turn down a distraught woman (or couple).

OCCASIONAL RULEBREAKERS

Most of the fifteen physicians interviewed who performed illegal abortions did so rarely, perhaps only once or several times during their pre-*Roe* careers. For example, Peter Smith was a family practitioner in a rural Southern town in the 1960s. In his practice local women continually begged him for abortions, and, as he put it, "I had absolutely no resources, no place I could send them, no advice I could give them." On one occasion, feeling so overwhelmed by the hopelessness of the patient before him (an indigent mother of four who had just left her abusive husband), he authorized a hysterectomy, although in fact such a procedure was not technically indicated. The younger physician assisting Smith during the operation at one point examined the patient, started to comment on the woman's pregnancy after feeling her uterus, and then, in Smith's words, "His eyes met mine, he nodded slightly, and didn't say anything else."

Ethel Bloom, also a family physician, was in practice in a large

East Coast city in the 1960s and had no experience whatsoever in abortion provision. Having experienced an unwanted pregnancy and the subsequent search for a qualified abortionist herself, however, she was enormously sympathetic to her patients and did everything she could to find them qualified providers. In one case, one of her closest friends – "we were like sisters" – came to her, begging for an abortion for her teenaged daughter, who was about to begin college. Bloom went to an ob/gyn in her network, a longstanding colleague on whom she could usually depend, but who for some reason this time refused to help. "I actually went down on my knees begging him – but I think he felt he had been doing too many lately, and his hospital had been breathing down his neck. I walked out of there shaking, and after I relaxed, it just came to me! I would say she had tested positive for rubella." (This was a period in which the hospitals in Bloom's city had just begun to approve rubella-indicated therapeutic abortions.) Bloom wrote a statement testifying that the young woman had been diagnosed as having rubella and sent her to the hospital with a request for an abortion. The chief of obstetrics in that hospital – "a known antiabortionist" – called Bloom and said to her, "If that patient really doesn't have rubella, you're going to be in trouble." Bloom responded, "Fine, retest her." She apparently won this staring-down match, because the procedure was done without a retest. (As she explained, in that period the test was more cumbersome and costly, and she simply took the risk that the doctor would not order another test.)

After this ruse proved successful, over the next several years until the *Roe* decision, Bloom successfully used the same technique with about eight other patients, always being careful to refer them to different doctors. Needless to say, the trustworthiness of patients was a major consideration for Bloom, given that she was obviously lying on their behalf. Bloom explained that those for whom she made such referrals were longstanding patients in her practice, where trust had already been established. She further stated her feeling that to undergo some risk on behalf of her patients was her obligation as a physician. "That's part of the practice of medicine . . . you do what you feel is necessary to insure the safety of your patients."

Sheldon Rothstein, a physician in practice in the New York area in the 1950s and 1960s, did not consider himself, in retrospect, a provider of illegal abortions. He nonetheless was very sympathetic to his patients and worked closely with a number of illegal abortionists, offering his patients both referrals and back-up services. Occasionally, however, he crossed the line and surreptitiously took part in the abortion itself.

> There was a nice immigrant doctor over in Jersey City, Dr. Ludwig [not his real name]. He was a pediatrician. Why he felt he needed the money, I don't know, but he did criminal abortions and he had a school principal who was pregnant, and he tried to abort her two or three times and he kept failing and didn't know why and finally he sent her to me. . . .
> The reason he never did the abortion, she had this large ovarian tumor which he mistook for the uterus. He never harmed her but he never aborted her. . . . I admitted her to my hospital with a diagnosis of twisted ovarian cyst, which was not quite accurate because it wasn't twisted, but it was a genuine ovarian tumor and I did a D. & C. and completed the abortion he had started and I did a laparotomy and removed her ovarian tumor.

When asked at this point in the interview how he felt about performing an abortion himself, Rothstein replied with a telling distinction: "I didn't *do* an abortion. I completed what he had started. The pathological diagnosis was incomplete abortion."

Joe Davidson recounted a story of colluding with nurses to perform a clandestine abortion in a hospital operating suite in the middle of the night. Davidson, an African-American, was the first member of his family to finish college. He was in his second year of an obstetrics/gynecology residency in a large Southern hospital when a fellow resident—"my best friend, my bosom buddy"—begged Davidson to perform an abortion on a nurse he had impregnated.

> She was an Operating Room nurse and she had colleagues on duty at night. . . . Her best girlfriend was on duty from midnight to seven, so we arranged it on a night when we knew nobody else would be around. . . .
> The thing that worried us, what if there was an emergency that came through the E.R.? What we did was keep in touch the whole night with

the E.R. We asked before we started if there was potential surgery that
they were going to send us . . . and we checked around on all the floors
and it looked as if it was going to be a quiet evening. And we knew it
wouldn't take that long. And we did it under a local . . . a paracervical
block. And she was about seven or eight weeks pregnant and I just did a
sharp curettage.

Several of those interviewed recalled incidents from an earlier
era when apparently it was possible to violate abortion laws more
flagrantly. Lionel Geiser, a California physician, had worked in an
Army hospital during World War II, where many of the nurses
needed abortions and a sympathetic pathologist kept as part of his
supplies a block of tissue that showed hyperplasia. "When an abortion came through, they threw the tissue away and cut a section from
this block and labeled it as hyperplasia, and so it was never recorded
as an abortion."[1]

Thomas Darrow, who presently provides abortions – with much
local opposition – in a highly conservative town in the South, was told
by a local colleague of the seemingly simpler period of abortion delivery that preceded *Roe* there.

One of the older doctors in town, he's retired now, told me about a small
private hospital run by a doctor and his son. . . . He said he could remember when a D. & C. in a private hospital was $25, including surgeon's
fees, anesthesia, room, and that included the abortion. . . . That private
hospital here in town was doing illegal abortions for a number of years
in the thirties till the sixties. . . . There was just one doctor on the staff,
this was *his* hospital. . . . He took the X-rays, he read the X-rays, he read
the tissue for pathology, did the pathology himself. . . . The people that
worked there were utterly devoted to him. He could do no wrong. Very
much like the situation in *Cider House Rules*.[2]

REGULAR RULEBREAKERS

Daniel Fieldstone. Daniel Fieldstone's pattern of providing illegal
abortions was probably the most typical of mainstream physicians
who did so before legalization. That is, he quietly performed abortions only on certain private patients with whom he had a special
relationship.

Fieldstone came from the New York area, the son of an obstetrician-gynecologist. He was a resident at Mount Sinai Hospital in the 1950s under Alan Guttmacher and thus was exposed early in his training to a variety of innovations in reproductive health. "I was in the right place at the right time." In addition to abortion reform, liberalized sterilization and birth control policies were part of Gutt-macher's agenda at Mount Sinai.[5] As Fieldstone recalled this heady, and controversial, atmosphere:

> We were also looking at the whole question of fertility in the 1950s. The abortion issue is only one part of it, although it's been portrayed as a single issue. Mount Sinai was much more notorious for its sterilization regulations, which looking backwards, were incredibly terrible, but at the time struck everyone as very liberal. There was the "rule of thirty" – you had to have six kids, living, by the time you were thirty, five by age thirty-five, four by age forty, or have had three C-sections, and you had to have the permission of your husband, or if you were separated, he had to have been gone seven years. . . . Those were the most liberal regulations in the country for elective sterilization, and we were sterilizing hundreds of Hispanics, blacks, poor women, who up to that time were having children every year. So six under thirty seemed like a big deal, but we had a lot of people who qualified.

Fieldstone commented on birth control at Mount Sinai. "We had a contraceptive clinic, a jammed contraceptive clinic, at a time when it was illegal to provide contraceptives in municipal hospitals. We were fitting diaphragms when women could die in a municipal hospital over a lack of contraception. So it all sort of hung together. Gutt-macher really was a descendant of Margaret Sanger in terms of his thinking. Which was of course that women had the right to control the number of children they wanted."

It was in this atmosphere that Fieldstone received training in the techniques of performing abortions, as well as a positive image of the abortion provider.

> Mount Sinai was virtually the only hospital in New York City that had a therapeutic abortion committee at that time and that allowed therapeutic abortions. Now in other places, you just died. . . . "Abortion" was such

a dirty word then . . . and "abortionist" was such a dirty word, it was just one step above a pervert, or child abuser. . . . It was incredible, to be called an abortionist in the 1950s, you were the scum of the earth . . . and in fact, the only time you ever saw the word "abortionist," it would be something like, "Bits of body found in Queens sewer traced to abortionist's office, who said he panicked when she died and he chopped her up and threw her down the sewer."[4]

Encouraged by Guttmacher and others at Mount Sinai, Fieldstone began what would become a career-long academic interest in abortion and undertook demographic research on the incidence of illegal abortion. This academic research soon became joined with political involvement in the movement, then emerging in New York state, to legalize abortion. "I had been working on this research for a number of years; it was part of the effort to assist the reform movement in getting a model abortion law passed, . . . but I was always more of a medical activist."

Fieldstone's attendance at the 1968 Hot Springs conference, sponsored by the Association for the Study of Abortion, was particularly important in giving him a sense of belonging to a professional community that was preparing for legal abortion. "That meeting . . . really changed everything. They brought together what we knew about incidence and effects of criminal abortion, what the effects of legalization were, and what was known then about techniques." Like the other physicians at the conference, whose hospital-based abortion experience was limited to the D. & C. method, Fieldstone was particularly struck by the display of the vacuum suction machine, which promised a far safer method of first trimester abortion. "The suction was an eye opener, it was such a superior technique – it shocked us."

In the early 1960s, Fieldstone for a time joined the private practice of his father, in the New York metropolitan area. There he gained his first experience in providing illegal abortions.

My father had always very quietly taken care of his own patients who had undesired pregnancies. He did do a few abortions. It was a very effective way, and you could get away with it unquestionably, as long as you didn't do it as a business. You would see them in the office, and use one of our biopsy instruments to create some bleeding and send them to the hospital as an incomplete abortion [where either of the Fieldstones then would complete the procedure]. So he took care of his own practice but he never took care of anybody else. I did the same. We never said anything about it, and we didn't charge any more for it, we didn't announce it, and we didn't take care of anybody else. It was a quiet, not particularly courageous act.

Fieldstone went on to explain why he and his father were so selective. "I wasn't going to be on the receiving end of the underground, dealing with hundreds of women coming for abortions and throwing my career and my license up for grabs."

In this statement (which was echoed by others in this study who also selectively offered abortions to private patients), the fear seemed to be not only of the potential number of abortion seekers, but also of their status as strangers.

Dad had been practicing in the same location in the Bronx since 1935. By the time I got there he was taking care of the daughters of the women he delivered in the 1930s. Before I left, he was taking care of their granddaughters. There really weren't too many strangers in that practice. So we didn't take much risk by dealing with people we didn't know. The biggest risk we took is we'd start one, and somehow or another they'd bleed to death or they'd get a super infection and get angry at us. It would have been a problem. But litigation wasn't as scary then as it is now.

"Risk management" then, for Fieldstone and his father, was a function both of dealing only with trusted longtime patients and of keeping volume down. As Fieldstone said, "Spontaneous abortion was pretty common; it's always going to be about 15 percent of your practice, so if you raised it to 20 percent, who would know? Nobody sat there at the end of the year and said, 'Daniel Fieldstone did x deliveries this year and y abortions.' Now if we had made a business of it, that would have been different."

Yet, as Fieldstone conceded, even some of those who did make a "business" of illegal abortion managed to avoid prosecution. A colleague at Mount Sinai Hospital was a case in point. "Everyone knew that Gene was doing [illegal] abortions. He was way out of range; you know, he had many abortions, very few deliveries. Nobody bothered him. That man went through his whole career without being hassled. He was the society abortionist. It proved that for enough money you could get away with anything. He was doing it at Sinai, at Doctors' Hospital, and a couple of small private hospitals."

When asked to speculate on Gene's motivations, Fieldstone responded, "I don't know how he got into it in the first place. He was a sweet, kind, and dear man. Very nice fellow. Maybe he wasn't the greatest gynecologist I ever saw and wasn't that comfortable with big stuff. And maybe he found a niche in life. Or maybe something moved him, I don't know." Yet, though Gene was clearly involved in abortion provision as a "business," in contrast to the Fieldstones' very occasional "service" to their clients, the former, in Fieldstone's view, most emphatically did not qualify as a "criminal abortionist . . . the kind you saw who were alcoholics, addicts, gamblers, sleaze bags . . . who would pick women up or their aides picked them up and blindfolded them and took them to a motel and all those ghastly stories."

Finally, like virtually everyone else interviewed for this study, Fieldstone commented on the unfairness of the situation that prevailed before the 1970s:

> Basically, the wealthy woman had access to a legitimate doctor. Occasionally she had to go overseas, but most of the time, if you had money, you'd find somebody, somebody reputable. By the 1960s, it wasn't any great problem because I could call up two of my psychiatrist friends and say to the patient, "You go over there and tell them you're going to commit suicide and for $100 apiece they'll write you a letter and that's that." We went to the committee in the hospital with those letters and that was it. Also, there was this handbook by Pat Maginnis; it taught you how to fake a suicide attempt . . . what you should say to a psychiatrist to convince him you're suicidal.[5] If you had the money, you could do it. The catch was, if you were fifteen years old, you couldn't do it. If you were black and poor, you couldn't do it. They ended up in our hospital emergency rooms.

Simon Ross. As discussed in the previous chapter, Simon Ross's experiences on a Native American reservation and in Korea were decisive in developing his commitment to fertility control, including his decision to provide illegal abortions. This decision involved a difficult break with his family traditions and, especially, his church.

> My dad was a physician in public health, and my mother had a couple of years of college. They were very conservative, very involved in their church. I was brought up to go to church twice on Sundays. I was very active in religious groups in medical school, like the Inner Varsity Christian Fellowship. So I had a very strong religious background. I wasn't a fanatic . . . but I was strongly religious. And I felt the solution to God's problems, in the world, was through faith – through faith in God we'd find a way to solve these problems. I became convinced, after I was on an Indian reservation and in Korea, that God wasn't going to solve all our problems. We've got to solve them ourselves. And that was it.

After Ross returned to the United States from Korea in 1966, he entered a large university in the Midwest to pursue advanced training in public health. "I decided to get my master's in maternal and child health and see what I could do to interest the maternal and child health people in the problem of family planning. There was very little interest then. I started going to the city of Chicago, visiting health clinics – talking to nurses, patients, and doctors about birth control. They kicked me out and told me never to come back."

Ultimately, however, Ross did find a compatriot in the African-American community who shared his commitment to making birth control available to the underserved. "I ended up, finally, in a black church in a working-class suburb. This minister wanted the clinic, and it started in the church basement with an all-black staff. . . . We offered pills, condoms, and I also offered IUDs and vasectomies." One of Ross's primary concerns was to avoid the high failure rate of IUDs that he had seen in his work in Korea. He tried, unsuccessfully, to innovate a more effective IUD. "The pregnancy rate was directly related to the amount of irritation to the uterus. The more irritation to the uterus, the fewer pregnancies. The most effective devices were those that caused the most symptoms. Women with the ones that didn't cause symptoms – the 'happy users' – those were the women who got pregnant. So I was getting pregnancies among the women there who had used the IUD, and I talked to the minister, and we decided, together, to go ahead and terminate the pregnancies of those women who wanted to."

While in Korea, Ross had observed a method of first trimester abortion that involved injecting saline solution into the uterus. He initially hesitated about using it in the church clinic.

> I was very wary about injecting saline. I was thinking, what if you get that into the bloodstream or something like that. . . . It would be so much easier if you could insert an IUD, and say they got pregnant using an IUD. There would be less legal risk. I tried a few IUDs, knowing they were pregnant, but it didn't work, it didn't terminate the pregnancies. I finally went back to saline. The Korean doctors were right. They didn't get infections. The women would spontaneously abort within three to five days. . . . I used an [IUD] inserter, and just a 25-cc syringe. I put it through the cervix, in the uterus, and slowly injected, over a period of five to ten minutes, 25 ccs of 25 percent saline. Very slowly. They would cramp some, but not severely. I'd leave them on the table for another five minutes and pick them up. I thought some would leak out, but it never did. . . . The mechanics of it are so simple. It dehydrates the placenta and the conception . . . so it's expelled.

Though in the several years he provided abortions in the church clinic, Ross did not have any run-ins with law enforcement, he did have some conflict with his university. "The Dean of the School of Public Health heard about it and called me in and told me I had to quit. He said I was the biggest troublemaker in the school. . . . I just let him yell at me. He has completely changed now [to a pro-choice position], which is interesting." Nevertheless, in spite of his abortion activity, Ross's other work was apparently valued by his institution, coinciding as it did with a burgeoning national interest in family planning. "Someone from the National Foundation came around [to the School of Public Health] and said that they had a lot of money to give to family planning. It was starting to be a big thing. Are you doing anything in family planning? The Dean said, 'Oh yeah. We've got one doctor, one crazy doctor who has got this clinic down in a church basement.' They sent off these Foundation people to check me. They came down there, in this basement, and watched me do vasectomies and insert IUDs."

Besides providing abortions in the church clinic, Ross very selectively offered abortions to people in his personal network, as well as to some of his private patients. "I was also doing some for friends . . . just very close friends. I did two or three in a period of two years. When they had gotten someone pregnant, I would help them out. I would actually go to the woman's house or apartment and just insert the 25 ccs of saline, no problems." It is interesting to note that those whom Ross did the abortion "for" were his male friends; a number of the other male providers of illegal abortion in this study similarly reported that their primary motivation was "helping out a buddy," though compassion for the pregnant woman was certainly not lacking. Ross also reported that he performed abortions, again very selectively, on patients in his private practice whose contraceptive, usually an IUD, had failed.

Ross reported a very high degree of success with this saline method. "I never had a problem once with this technique, ever. I did hundreds. I had to repeat maybe one or two out of a hundred, but no hemorrhages. I never had to have a D. & C. done on them, no infections." He expressed puzzlement that this method had apparently not been more in use in this country both before and after *Roe*. "I thought to myself, why is it that women always insert things like catheters and foreign objects in their uterus, when all they'd have to do is this?" The lack of knowledge of this technique made him hesitate to use it openly when abortion was legal, in spite of the success he had. "It [saline injection] wasn't accepted and I was afraid. If I did have a complication, legally I might have a problem because everyone else was doing D. & C.'s and having good success. . . . I never felt comfortable writing it up [experience with this method] because it was illegal when I was doing them. How are you going to report it? So science was held back."

Although all of those interviewed who provided illegal abortions used sliding scales to set fees, and occasionally performed abortions *gratis*, Ross was among the few who never charged a patient for an abortion, neither in the church clinic nor among his friends and patients. This policy stemmed in part from legal caution, in part from some ambivalence about making money from abortion work. Asked to reflect on how much fear he had felt at the time about police detection, he responded, "No, I didn't feel scared. . . . I'm not sure why. One thing I felt, I was not charging for it. I was not making money on it. I thought, both on a personal basis and on a legal basis, I would be on better ground if I did not charge." Elsewhere in the interview, Ross contrasted his feelings about abortion work before *Roe* and after, and acknowledged a certain nostalgia for the former period – "when it wasn't done for the money" and he could feel himself to be a "idealistic activist."

The ambivalence that Ross felt about *being paid* for performing abortions did not seem to reflect an ambivalence about abortion *per se.* As he reflected about his abortion practice, particularly in the period of illegality when abortions were rare, "I, as a medical doctor, got tremendous personal medical satisfaction out of doing them. I felt there was nothing that I could do with my background and training that would help people more, medically and socially . . . that would [contribute to] the health and happiness of their families, if I didn't give abortions. The time they spent looking around for an abortion and nobody else wanting to do them." The hesitation expressed about being paid for abortion work – expressed strongly by Ross and to a lesser degree by some other interviewees – is an interesting part of the story of abortion provision in the United States, and I will return to it in the final chapter.

Irving Goodman. Unlike Simon Ross, whose commitment to abortion provision meant overcoming a very conservative social and religious background, Irving Goodman had a number of influences in his life that made such a commitment seem almost inevitable. He was born in 1926 in a large East Coast city to Russian Jewish immigrants, with, as he put it, socialism and the pursuit of social justice the "religion" of his upbringing. The political consciousness he developed in childhood contributed to his decision, many years later, to offer illegal abortions. "It was definitely a political statement . . . because the rich could get it. This was pissing me off, really. Because, if you had enough money, I knew they could get the damn thing done. But these people [served by him] were not rich, they were working class."

But there were personal issues as well in his early life that pushed him toward eventually providing illegal abortions. As a young teenager, he learned of an abortion tragedy in his own family. "My mother was orphaned when she was twelve. And I have some beautiful pictures of my grandmother, whom I never had met. The most beautiful woman I'd ever seen, in a picture. And I found out that she died of an illegal abortion. And my mother was twelve, the oldest of five kids. And I began to hear stories like that, more and more." Most fundamental to Goodman's future decision was his own harrowing experience, at the age of eighteen, recounted in chapter 3, with his future wife's poorly performed illegal abortion.

As a medical student, Goodman became very interested in the medical aspects of abortion and wrote his major research paper on the subject. As an intern and resident in a large West Coast hospital in the mid-1950s, predictably he confronted many women suffering from the effects of illegal abortion. Early in his experience there, he witnessed an abortion-caused death that had eerie similarities to the situation of his mother and grandmother. "There was a thirty-one-year-old Mexican-American woman, with five children. She died in septic shock, with her family around her, with a prolonged endotoxic death situation."

Unlike the others who became involved in illegal abortion, Goodman was surrounded by collegial fellow residents who almost universally shared his frustration with restrictive abortion laws. His frustration was seemingly shared by their superiors as well. "I'm not too sure that the supervisors weren't on our side either. Because these patients were just taking up beds and occupying our time and everything else. To get them healthy was the goal of everybody. But I don't remember any real negatives about abortion, other than statements about the person who induced it on the outside – the abortionist, that 'nasty person,' who had created all these problems for us."

Goodman and his fellow residents not only had massive experience with completing abortions started by others, some started to push the hospital rules to the limit by performing abortions on patients with the most marginal of indications. This rule bending, if not outright rule breaking, could only occur because of the collusion of like-minded residents. As Goodman recalled, "I would be more in-

clined to . . . not necessarily falsify, but to project my eye into seeing
something further along than someone else would. If the cervix was
starting to dilate, you could [legally] do it . . . and I was not the only
one doing that. . . . One of us would say to the other, 'She has to be
emptied. You're on call tonight.' 'Is she dilating?' 'Yeah, I can see it
from here.'"

The extensive experience Goodman gained from completing septic abortions that had been started outside the hospital; from performing hospital-approved abortions, e.g., on patients with rubella;
and from performing the quasi-legal abortions mentioned above
made him feel confident that he could provide complete abortions
outside the hospital. As Simon Ross had, Goodman did his first such
abortion at the request of his best friend, whose wife was experiencing an unwanted pregnancy.

In recollecting his first illegal abortions, Goodman conceded that
he had displayed bravado and perhaps overconfidence in his medical
skills at the time. "I wasn't going to take a chance on starting one in
the office and then sending the woman to the hospital. It was obvious
that the operation itself could be done quite easily. You needed proper
anesthetic, you didn't want to hurt anybody. So I did it in the home. . . .
I used the back of the chair for stirrups – a very simple method, put a
pillow over the back of upright chairs on the edge of the bed. And you
created an operating room, just like the old people [veteran physi-
cians] used to do deliveries. It's very simple."

When asked what kind of anesthetic he had used, Goodman replied, "Well, at times I used the saddle block anesthesia, being too
stupid to know that it was probably too dangerous. But I was very adept at using that. And then when I got frightened from doing that, not
because of anything I did, but the intellectual understanding that this
is probably not a good idea, then I gave the patient three grains of Sec-
onal, one hundred of Demerol, and some scopolamine. I was in my
third year of residency and I had access to all this stuff in my hospital. . . . I was probably betting my skills, because for me, I felt there
was no problem. It was very simple. Even though I was doing another
sharp curettage. Remember, I had a lot of experience with the
septics."

Goodman estimates that he performed approximately thirty-five or so out-of-hospital abortions over a five-year period. Initially, these abortions were restricted to people close to Goodman and his wife. "We had friends and relatives flying out from the East Coast. . . . My wife would inform me, 'So and so is pregnant, and they just can't afford another kid.' And I would say, 'Fine, tell her to come out and we'll do it.'" Goodman's fees ranged from nothing, for those who could not afford to pay or for family members and close friends, to a usual fee of $200. "The maximum I was ever given was someone who wanted to give me $600. And this was a very rich spoilt lady, who was really angry at her mother. She said, 'My mother can afford to shell out a lot more and you are going to charge me that.' I said, 'Okay, fine.'"

But Goodman found it was very difficult – once he became known as someone willing to perform abortions – to restrict his clientele. One reason that he found it difficult to confine himself to friends was his astonishment at how easy the whole process seemed, technically. "You start doing it, and you get good at it, and you feel good. Then you start saying, 'Well, here's a patient, this is someone that you know very well.'" So Goodman began to do abortions for selected patients, which in turn led to requests from friends of the patients. "A patient says, 'Look, there's my best friend, or my cousin, and she's been looking around, and she has to pay $1,000' [for an illegal abortion], and that's silly. So I said, 'It shouldn't cost that much – $200, or something like that.' So you get sucked into helping somebody and they give you a little money for that.'"

Although Goodman never had any confrontation with the police over his illegal abortion activity, what made him stop was the enormous demand for abortions and the seeming impossibility of keeping it private. "What I found out, over a period of time, which made me back off from this, was that if you did it for one person, they told someone else. . . . You could not control that in any way, shape, or form. And that was the time I said to myself, 'This is idiotic.'" Goodman's wife, though initially supportive of his performing illegal abortions selectively, had become increasingly concerned about the growing demands on him, and with her encouragement, Goodman stopped.

Though Goodman's primary motivation for providing illegal

abortions was compassion for those – like his wife and himself – who
had faced an unwanted pregnancy, he candidly acknowledged other
psychological factors. Reflecting – twenty-five years after the fact – on
his mindset at the time, Goodman said: "You have to understand,
now, I'd probably be struck by the magnitude of the risk I took. . . . At
that time, I was young and didn't think it was that much of a risk. . . .
With me, it was just sliding into it from one stage to another. And then
certain things occurred . . . you did more. And the more you did, the
more relaxed you were about it. There was a sense of excitement
about it . . . like some people climb mountains, like some people do
scuba diving, and some people are risk-takers. . . . It was a turn-on.
This whole thing of making, of thinking and planning and everything else. There was a kind of excitement."

David Bennett. David Bennett is distinguished from the other
respondents (except one) in this subsample of fifteen providers of illegal abortion in that he ultimately made the decision to offer an
abortion to all who requested one. Although the small number of participants in this study dictates caution in drawing conclusions, it is
nonetheless intriguing that Bennett and the other provider of abortion on request, Henry Morgentaler (whose case will be discussed
next) were the two interviewees who most explicitly tied their decision to perform abortions to their earlier involvement in progressive
political movements.

Bennett was born and raised in the rural Southwest. While drawing away from the fundamentalist Southern Baptism that surrounded him in his family and community, he was, as a teenager,
deeply interested in the philosophical dimensions of religion. "Religion was a primary intellectual outlet for me. . . . I was interested in,
how do we live our lives with a sense of fairness? . . . What is just?"
His first awareness of the issues of abortion and unwanted pregnancy
was as an adolescent.

> Something happened when I was in high school. That's when I can
> trace back when I really began to accept the possibility of being
> involved in abortions in the future. . . . There was a young woman that
> was kept outside of the group. I came to find out that she had a child and
> had not been married, and before this event occurred, she had been pop-

ular and belonged to clubs, was a good singer. She was no longer allowed to participate in anything – she could come to class and that was it. This seemed very unfair to me. . . . I knew other boys and girls in the high school were engaging in sexual activities. It was rumored that there was someone who would do abortions for $500 (which in 1953 was a tremendous sum of money), so if you had enough money there would be a different outcome, but here she was. . . . It had a very profound effect on me.

In medical school in the early 1960s, Bennett received some training in abortion which, typical for that period, centered on dealing with complications of illegal abortions as well as learning to complete spontaneous abortions (miscarriages). The message Bennett received from professors about abortion was unequivocally negative – both the physicians who provided this service and the women who sought it were to be condemned. Also, like many others interviewed for this study, Bennett was urged to report to the police any women who came to the emergency room suspected of having had an illegal abortion. "I was naive. Once I reported someone who had an illegal abortion, the police came and questioned her, she reported who did it, and they went to arrest this person, the woman who induced the abortion, and filed charges against her. That was the last one I ever reported." Remorse over this incident increased Bennett's compassion for those seeking abortions as well as for those who provided them, even if their competence was questionable. "There were many unethical people – 'butchers' – and those who did it primarily for gain, but I think in those days there were [also] those – more often women, usually nurses – who did it in good conscience, and did what they knew how to do, and often they got bad results. But I don't think they were all bad people."

Bennett's actual involvement in abortion began several years later, in 1967, when he was just establishing a family practice in the small town in which he had been raised. Pressures to become involved with abortion came from two overlapping groups with which he was then involved: the local Unitarian Church, a denomination that Bennett had joined as a medical student, and the "movement" – a loose confederation of local groups involved in the key social issues of that period: civil rights, opposition to the Vietnam War, and newly emerging feminism.

The Unitarian clergy in Bennett's area had just become involved with the state affiliate of the Clergy Consultation Service on Abortion. The CCS, originally started in New York in 1967, eventually grew to include some fourteen hundred clergy in two dozen states. These groups made abortion referrals both inside the United States and abroad, before legalization. Before 1971 all referrals were to reliable illegal practitioners of abortion; after 1971, the clergy referred to clinics in New York state and elsewhere where abortion laws had been repealed or substantially liberalized. The CCS chapters all followed the same basic model. Women seeking abortions would call a phone number listed by the local CCS, after which they would then be guided to a clergyperson who would meet with them personally. Women were required to bring to this meeting a statement ascertaining the fact and length of their pregnancy. (For women whose own physicians refused to cooperate by providing this statement – fearing it would implicate them in the abortion – or for those who had no private physician, the CCS would refer to local physicians who would provide such documentation.) The woman would then be offered personal counseling, if desired, about her decision to abort, be given an explanation of the procedure, and be provided with the name and fee of an abortion provider. (The CCS decided to refer only to licensed physicians, preferably ob/gyns.) All physicians to whom the CCS chapters referred had been screened by clergy or their associates. Physicians were screened on the basis of their standard procedures – for example, the CCS's medical advisors deemed those who used general anesthesia in their offices too risky – as well as their overall demeanor, the appearance of their offices, and, especially, their reasonableness about fees. Furthermore, the participating clergy asked the women they counseled to give them feedback on the abortion experience – and according to the organization's founders, a surprising 40 percent did offer such postabortion evaluations. The most typical reason for dropping a physician from a CCS referral list was his or her refusal to set what were considered reasonable fees. (The original New York chapter, in 1967, set $600 as the highest acceptable fee.) No fees were ever charged for counseling and referral. In spite of the thousands of referrals which were made between 1967 and 1973 (about one hundred thousand, without any fatalities among the women referred, according to its founders), there was only minimal legal interference in these services. Two clergy – one minister, one rabbi – were arrested for offering such referrals, but prosecution in each case was ultimately dropped.[6]

The Unitarian clergy in Bennett's state, who had encountered him during his medical school days and later at summer retreats, sensed his sympathy with the abortion issue and urged that he offer illegal abortions, or short of that, that he be willing to serve as a back-up physician for women who received abortions out of the country or from local "underground" practitioners.

Pressures from Bennett's political comrades, in the loosely organized "movement" circles in his region, were more intense and personal.

> At that time, we would have many sessions where we would talk about "What kind of world did we want?" and there were many women there. . . . It became obvious that many felt it wasn't a fair world for women. . . . The consequences of sexual activity can be so devastating to a woman, and to a man it could even be a source of pride or prestige. . . . He could go right on with his college career, and a pregnancy can interrupt her life. Her life is radically and drastically changed, which didn't apply to the man. If she should find herself pregnant, for whatever reason, she should have the choice of terminating that pregnancy. And once I came to that position, it became harder and harder for me to resist doing what I felt I could do.

Bennett underwent a period of extensive soul-searching with his wife, clergy friends, lawyer, and other close associates. He then made the decision to offer abortions to all those who sought them. Part of this soul-searching meant considering the possibility of a prison sentence. "I was talking with a friend of mine, who taught at a Baptist seminary. I said, 'Well, if I go to prison, there's a lot of books I want to read.' You understand, this was very naive. In retrospect, prison is not time off to go to the library. It was part of a lot of inner deception. I think it was one way of controlling some of the fear and apprehension I had."

Bennett began to integrate abortion provision into his general practice, at first accepting referrals only through the Clergy Consultation Service. He recalled one of his most memorable cases.

I had a minister from San Antonio who used to send people to me. One day he called me to say a woman was coming on the bus to see me. . . . It was kind of vague, when she was going to come, if she was really going to come, but he was saying she might show up. . . . Sure enough one day she did. This was a Latin American woman in her late forties who had ridden from San Antonio, Texas to my little town where no one had ever spoken any Spanish. That's not true now, but at that time, she was coming into a foreign world. She spent the night in the rest room of the hospital, because she knew they stayed open all night. So she slipped in, and hid in the rest room. . . . I still don't know how she got there.

So she shows up at my office. Now I don't speak any Spanish at that time. Through sign language I finally realized, this is the woman they were talking about, from San Antonio. I finally realized she wanted an abortion. I asked her how she was getting back. So she pulled out a bus ticket. She also pulled out her purse, and she had a dirty crumpled wallet, and dropped it in my hand, and it had a five dollar bill in it. . . . And I'm just so moved that she has got herself here, it seemed incredible to me. She came with no money, just faith. I mean she's come all this way with just a dirty crumpled five dollar bill to pay for an abortion. I wanted to give her the money back. At the same time, I didn't want to offend her sense of dignity. I know she stayed at the hospital rest room, this is all the money she's got. I looked in her purse, she's got these tortillas in her purse, that's what she's living on – these tortillas. So I somehow managed to say to her that I would like to provide the service free, that she so honored me by making the great effort to get here, that I would like to provide the abortion for her free, if that was all right with her. I knew everything was all right, because a big smile came on her face, she reached out and took the five dollar bill and put it back in her purse. Those were the kinds of situations I saw then.

When he first began providing abortions Bennett would induce an abortion in his office and then send the woman to the hospital emergency room where she was to claim she was having a miscarriage. On occasion, particularly when he first started, Bennett would perforate a patient's uterus or other complications would occur. In such situations, it obviously was impossible for the woman to claim she was miscarrying, and Bennett had to hope that she would not reveal who had performed her abortion. "You just had to trust them to lie for you and refuse to tell. It was a terrible situation. And these women understood that, they wanted the service and they believed we'd done the best we could. They knew that if I went to jail, none of them were going to get this abortion." Commenting on the fact that no injured patient had ever betrayed him in a hospital, Bennett speculated about the special bond that could develop between provider and patient in the era of illegality. As he put it, "I had to trust her – after all, she was trusting her life and health to me."

Bennett soon grew dissatisfied with his method of starting an abortion then having the patient report to a hospital emergency room to have it completed. "These women are going to all kinds of hospitals. They are bleeding and cramping, they may get infections, they've got all these potential complications. They've got a big hospital bill. Sometimes they have police hassling them. This is just no way to do this. There must be a better way. That's when I decided I was going to order the instruments, I was going to do it [the entire procedure]. I was going to complete the surgery in such a way that the woman could bear it. I had already been entering the cervix, I knew I could go in with instruments and get into the uterus."

When Bennett decided to escalate his already illegal practice by offering complete abortions, he realized he would be intensifying the risks. First, he needed to order the instruments necessary to do a complete D. & C.: "I just called and ordered the instruments. . . . I called the detail man who serviced me; he brought over a pretty good instrument catalog, and I ordered all these instruments, dilators, curettes and all the instruments you need in the hospital. It was scary. . . . This detail man, he knew by the order that you don't order these instruments. . . . It was obvious why I was ordering them. But I did it." Bennett's abortion practice became much easier, technically, when suction machines became available around 1968, though again, the actual act of ordering the machine was nerve-wracking.

Predictably, Bennett's decision to offer illegal abortions created problems for him. First, though he had done a few abortions in the hospital while a medical student and intern, he was now engaged in full-scale abortion work without any colleagues with whom he could consult. Recalling the isolation he felt during that period, and his reluctance to confer with peers, he said: "I had no one to talk to, because I didn't want to jeopardize them. . . . I had the feeling that if anything happened, I didn't want them to be in a position of testifying against me. Some of them were people I knew, if I told them, they'd have to lie under oath, and I didn't want people to be put in that position."

Reconciling the flow of abortion patients with the rest of his practice was another problem for Bennett. Although initially he intended to restrict abortion patients to those who came to him via the Clergy Consultation Service, this soon proved impossible, as abortion seekers came to him from all over and he felt incapable of turning them down. His abortion work grew in such volume that it overwhelmed other aspects of his small-town family practice: "There were too many abortion patients coming and it was hard, because it was becoming apparent to most patients from town that there were strangers in the waiting room. And also, if I did have someone in pain, they would hear them crying out and wonder what was going on." Thus, with considerable wistfulness, Bennett gave up his family practice and began to do abortions full time.

Security was of course a major concern for Bennett. Even before becoming involved in abortion, he had occupied a very visible, and ambiguous, position in his community. On the one hand, his father was a well-respected figure in local politics, and Bennett himself was active in various mainstream community activities, such as the school board. On the other hand, his involvement in "movement" activities was conspicuous in this highly conservative area. Summing up his rather anomalous position in town, Bennett said, "I was the guy who wore the black armband [to protest the Vietnam War] when I had lunch at the Rotary Club."

Bennett's already tenuous relationship with the local authorities, especially the police, became worse as his abortion traffic increasingly came from out of town. At one point, in fact, the local police suspected him of being a drug trafficker: "Cars and vans are coming into town, many with out-of-state plates. In this county people notice out-of-state plates. They [police] start following these cars. They think I'm in the drug business. . . . Most of these are young people. The boyfriend comes with them, they bring friends with them. . . . The young people in those days, they come in, they have the long hair, hippie clothes on, they're smoking marijuana and they come cruising into town for their abortion. The police just watch all this and pull them over." In one particularly nerve-wracking incident, an abortion patient whose boyfriend had been arrested by police as the couple were en route to the abortion rushed into Bennett's office and proceeded to flush some marijuana down the toilet, leaving Bennett terrified of an imminent police raid.

Blackmail attempts by patients were one of the greatest threats during this period. As Bennett put it, "I could have gone to the police and said, 'I'm going to do abortions today' – but unless someone were there to bring charges, they couldn't do a thing about it. But all you need is one patient unhappy, one bad outcome, and that's it. So every patient I saw in those days was a potential." In fact, out of the thousands of illegal abortions that Bennett performed before *Roe*, only one blackmail attempt was made (by the boyfriend of a patient). After considerable thought, Bennett decided he could not capitulate and simply refused to cooperate. "I told him to go to the police if he wanted. I said, 'The police know I'm doing abortions; sometimes they refer people to me.' I never heard from him again."

Given today's litigious climate and the overall atmosphere of distrust between many physicians and patients, it does seem remarkable that there were no more blackmail attempts against Bennett. Beyond the unquestionable fact of simple luck, other consideration help to explain this. First, most of Bennett's patients were prescreened by clergy working for the Consultation Service, where they were informed not only about the technical aspects of abortion but also about the risks that the cooperating physicians were undertaking. Second, the policies that Bennett himself adapted for his abortion practice also were conducive to a relationship of trust: he reduced or waived the fee in cases of financial need; he informed all patients that he would refund their fees if they were not satisfied with his service; and if any patient needed to be hospitalized after the procedure, Bennett would pay her bill.

It is also clear, in retrospect, that the abortion service that Bennett offered was quite different from that of many other abortion providers of that period (and indeed, of many practitioners today) – and this, too, may help to account for the loyalty of so many patients. Basically, Bennett quite early in his abortion career became committed to making the abortion a "positive experience" for the recipient. Initially, this meant trying to find ways to reduce the pain of the abortion: "It was the pain that bothered me. Women sometimes experienced excruciating pain. . . . I'm doing this for reasons of conscience and compassion and here I'm inflicting this terrible pain on women. . . . They would bite their lips till they bled." Bennett was experimenting with various kinds of local anesthetics but felt constrained from too much experimentation, given that his operations were totally removed from a hospital setting. He soon came to observe that the patients who came to him through the clergy consultation network as a whole suffered less pain than those who came from other referrals. "I began to ask the women who went to the ministers why they had less pain. They were less scared, they were more confident, . . . they had some issues they had talked about. Well, that led me from the pain medication to get on with relaxation techniques and hypnosis. I certainly became aware that fear was a major contributor to your reaction to the procedure."

Bennett's interest, developed in this pre-*Roe* era, in the related issues of pain management, relaxation techniques, and what would only later be known as "abortion counseling," would lead to a career-long interest in the woman's abortion experience (as opposed to the more narrow medical focus on the abortion procedure). As he later reflected on his mindset during his days as a provider of illegal abortions:

> I didn't want abortions to be simply the lesser of two evils. I wanted this to be a humane experience, but more than that . . . no matter how conflicted the woman might be, even feeling bad about herself . . . that she feel good about those providing the service . . . and perhaps we could

facilitate her feeling better about herself . . . and this could be a growth experience for her, that out of this she would have a sense of her own worth. If we provided services in a dignified way, respecting her as an individual, involving her in the process, then she could feel her own strength. So that's how we went from thinking of this as the lesser of two evils to a life-enhancing experience.

While Bennett received only one serious blackmail threat and was never formally charged by the police for performing abortions, his life nonetheless during the three years he offered abortions in his hometown was extremely stressful. Because of rumors about his abortion activity and his other controversial political activities, he and his family (which included three young children) constantly were harassed and began to receive physical threats. "It got very intense, it had the feeling of warfare, there was such controversy around. . . . We had some immigration cases, some civil rights cases going – we were sponsoring a music festival to raise money for some of these legal activities, and that caused a sellout of ammunition in town. I mean, we had to cancel the festival for fear some of them were going to get killed."

Bennett always felt the threat of possible arrest. "I got to this point, seeing a police car in my rearview mirror caused irrational fear." After three years of such pressure, he moved with his family to a large city, where he continued to perform illegal abortions for the next two years. He then moved to a nearby state, which by the early 1970s had considerably liberalized its abortion laws.

Henry Morgentaler. Unlike all the others interviewed for this book, who are based in the United States, Henry Morgentaler has spent his entire medical career in Canada, where he has been the single most influential medical activist on behalf of abortion reform in that country.[7] Though the Canadian abortion situation is somewhat different from that in the United States – most significantly, there has been no one legal decision with the force of the *Roe v. Wade* ruling in 1973 – Morgentaler's case is nonetheless relevant here for several reasons. After he began to openly perform illegal abortions, starting in 1968, he treated numerous women from the United States, including many who were sent to him by the Clergy Consultation Service. In his various court battles with the Canadian government, he has been supported by longstanding colleagues from the United States, such as Jane Hodgson, who has testified on his behalf on several occasions. Both before and after the *Roe* decision in the United States, Morgentaler has sustained professional relationships with U.S. abortion providers, and he has been instrumental in bringing Canadian colleagues into the National Abortion Federation, the leading organization of abortion providers in North America which is based in Washington, D.C.

Morgentaler was born in 1923 in Lodz, Poland into a highly political, secular Jewish family. "Socialism was the religion of our family." As a child, Morgentaler experienced much antisemitism from his Polish neighbors, ranging from beatings by local youths to manipulations of his grades by school authorities so that he would not outperform the non-Jewish students. With the coming of Naziism to Poland, Morgentaler's father, Josef, was arrested and subsequently killed. Eventually, the rest of the family was sent to concentration camps, where his mother and sister perished. Morgentaler and a younger brother survived six years in Dachau and Auschwitz.

After the war, Morgentaler studied medicine in Germany and Belgium. He moved to Canada in 1951 with his wife, also a concentration camp survivor, and completed his medical studies there. In one of the many anomalies that was to characterize Morgentaler's life in Canada, the Chancellor of the University of Montreal – a Catholic institution – who presented the new doctor with his diploma was later to become the Archbishop of Montreal. "He didn't know what kind of black sheep I would become later, but I didn't know that either. I didn't dream at the time of being involved in the abortion controversy."

After receiving a license to practice in Canada in 1955, Morgentaler started a family practice in a working-class section of Montreal. The abortion issue was not an overly pressing one for him in his early years of practice. He did however see a number of patients suffering from the aftereffects of illegal abortions, and recalled hospitalizing one of his patients who had almost died from such a procedure. He also wryly recollected, from his initial years of practice, a conversation with a senior physician. Morgantaler had raised the question of whether something could be done about the problem of illegal abortion, and his senior colleague replied, "Henry, don't touch this with a ten-foot pole. You'll be called an abortionist, they'll take your license away, you'll go to jail. This is a taboo subject."

Morgentaler periodically received requests from his patients for abortions, the overwhelming majority of which he would refuse. Over a twelve-year period from 1955 to 1967, he did perform a few illegal abortions: "maybe two or three cases, they were good patients for many years. . . . I felt scared but still I felt I had to help them, and they were very grateful and everything went fine. But I did it with a great deal of reluctance and a great deal of fear and anxiety that if something went wrong, I would really be in trouble."

Morgentaler's first significant political affiliation in Canada was with the Canadian Humanist Association. Joining such a group, as he saw it, was a direct outgrowth of his militantly secular upbringing. "I was brought up in an antireligious atmosphere. Religion was a dead weight . . . the acceptance of the status quo, the acceptance of injustice, the acceptance of inferior status, the acceptance of all kinds of indignities. I was brought up in a family which had broken away from all that. . . . The Jewish socialist movement was a complete break with the past – it affirmed human dignity. We don't accept the status quo just because religion says God wills it. But we have to do something to make society more just."

It was through the Humanist group that Morgentaler first became squarely engaged with abortion politics. In 1967, in response to the liberalization of abortion law in Great Britain, sectors of the Canadian medical community began to agitate for similar liberalization in Canada. Canada at the time had a highly restrictive abortion policy, in which the procedure was legal only to save the life of the mother. The Canadian government responded by establishing a parliamentary committee to study the abortion issue, and the Humanist Fellowship of Montreal decided to submit a brief. As Morgentaler was a physician, he soon was drawn into a leadership role, and he both researched and presented the Humanist brief to the Canadian Parliament in 1967.

Morgentaler acknowledges that initially he became politically engaged with abortion not out of a particular concern for "women's" issues, but by circumstance, as his Humanist group responded to developments in Canadian politics. "It just happened that these were women being discriminated against. If they had been men, with another issue, I could have put my energies into that too. It just happened to be women who were being denied fundamental human rights."

However, researching the abortion issue in depth was a radicalizing experience for Morgentaler, and he came to understand abortion in the larger context of two issues with which he already deeply resonated – social injustice and religious intolerance.

> I did the research . . . and here was a situation where women were discriminated against, exploited, were subjected to the danger of losing their lives, losing their fertility, and nobody was doing anything about it. A situation of tremendous injustice, and I said to myself, "Well, doctors usually go into medicine for humanitarian motives" (maybe more in Eastern Europe than in Canada or the United States). I went into medicine with very idealistic motives. Many doctors would go to countries in Africa and South America and subject themselves to the dangers of yellow fever, cholera, and what not. Some of them would even die, and they were taking enormous risks for humanity. Here in our own society, nobody was willing to take risks to help women with this kind of problem. It didn't make sense. And I researched it, and it seemed like it was religious prejudice.

In October 1967, Morgentaler presented to the Health Committee of the House of Commons the brief of the Humanist Fellowship of Montreal. This brief, endorsed by similar Humanist groups elsewhere in Canada, called for Canadian law to permit abortion on request. Though the Humanist recommendation was not followed, a new, slightly liberalized Canadian abortion law was passed in 1969 which permitted abortion, in hospitals only, upon the approval of a three-physician committee, in cases of threat to the life or health of the pregnant woman.

Morgentaler's high visibility on the abortion issue, both before Parliament and in other public forums, immediately brought him a stream of requests from all over Canada from pregnant women seeking abortions. Initially he refused all such requests. However, several factors led him to reconsider this decision. One was that the small pool of illegal abortionists whom he trusted and had used for referrals had dried up. "At the time . . . there was not a single doctor in Montreal who did good abortions. . . . I knew a doctor who was doing a reasonably good job, but he died in an accident. Another doctor who had done good work left the country, because of a court case. So there was nobody around."[8]

Already in a period of soul-searching, Morgentaler was also especially vulnerable at this time to wrenching stories of abortion-related injury and death. As he recalled, "What helped me [make the decision] was one terrible story about a woman, a mother of a three-year-old – I think she had broken up with her husband – and she asked her boyfriend to abort her. He used a bicycle pump, pumped air into her uterus, and she died from an embolism on the spot. So this guy was brought to court and he was crying and said, 'I didn't know, I was trying to help her, she wanted me to help.' But the story was such that if the woman had come to me – I know how to do a D. & C. – I could have helped her." This incident, and similar ones that came to Morgentaler's attention, heightened his sense of responsibility as a physician. "The image I had was that if you had a person drowning in the lake, and you were there, able to help that person just by extending your arm, everyone would do that, right? And in this particular case, would you do it, if it was, say, forbidden? . . . I told myself, 'Well, it would be a normal human gesture on my part to help.'"

A final contributing factor to Morgentaler's decision to provide illegal abortions was a growing sense of his own hypocrisy. "I started feeling like a preacher who doesn't practice what he preaches. I was talking about it [abortion] all the time, and finally a nurse in the hospital where I worked said to me, 'Dr. Morgentaler, you talk so much about it, why don't you do it?' She had chutzpah! I was taken aback. She was right. Because it wasn't good [to be] preaching something and having people come to me, and I was saying, 'I can't do it.' Where was the integrity? Finally I decided one day that I'm not going to refuse."

Thus in 1968 Henry Morgentaler began to openly provide abortions in his office in Montreal. He established this new service with two principles uppermost in his mind. "If I do it, I have to do it first of all with the safest procedure there is. . . . And the other principle was that no one would be refused an abortion because of inability to pay, because I knew that I would be accused of wanting to make a lot of money. So I set a reasonable fee, which had been set by another doctor who had done abortions in Canada, who seemed to be very nice – and that was $300." Later, as his abortion practice grew, Morgentaler enlisted the help of social service agencies in Montreal to help him set sliding-scale fees and also to help him establish guidelines for subsidized abortions for those unable to pay.

The enormous risk he was taking was very evident to him. Speaking of a colleague in British Columbia who had been convicted of providing abortions, Morgentaler said, "Well, this person only got three months, but his license was taken away of course, and he had a criminal record, and a possible punishment of life imprisonment was on the books. And the danger of course was that if a patient died by mischance, or there was an accident, which is always possible, I would . . . be ruined. That was actually my greatest worry, that the patient was going to die accidentally, and then I would not only be called a criminal, but an incompetent guy, someone who caused someone's death. . . . So it wasn't easy."

Having made the decision to offer abortions, Morgentaler sought counsel from a lawyer.

> I had the lawyer who I knew from the Civil Liberties Union where I was a director, and I said, "I started doing abortions and I intend to continue. I just want to ask you if you can give me some advice how not to be detected by the police." He said, "Well, my advice is not to do it." I said, "I'm doing it, I'm not going to stop. I want to know how to lower the chances of discovery and prosecution." He said, "Well, the best thing to do in that case is to not let anyone in with the patient and there would be no witnesses." I tried that for a day or two and then the women were anxious, and so were the husband, sister, the lover, etc. It was inhuman. So I disregarded my lawyer's advice, and I said, "What the hell." I allowed people to come in together and of course that reassured people.

In establishing his medical procedures, Morgentaler initially used the vacuum suction method, which was just at this period becoming widely known in England and North America. However, early in his abortion practice, a patient caused him to modify his methods. "I remember the first who had a complication. She called me from the hospital, she said, 'Doctor, I want to tell you that I had an abortion three days ago and I had a fever after that, and I had to go to the hospital and they told me it was incomplete and they had to do a D. & C., so I'm just calling to tell you that maybe you could improve your methods.' So I thanked her, and at that point I decided that just the suction wasn't enough, and I had to do a curettage on top of that. . . . So I started doing suction and curettage to make sure it was complete, and then I would re-suction." Morgentaler believes that he was the first doctor in North America to use this combined method of vacuum suction and curettage, now in wide use.[9]

Like David Bennett, the only other participant in this study who offered abortions to anyone who requested one, Morgentaler had a remarkable record of patient satisfaction and mutual trust. "If I didn't believe that it would work out, I wouldn't have done it. If I didn't trust people, I would not have let the lover, the mother, the sister come in with the patient, like my lawyer advised. But it has this opposite effect, when you trust people, ordinarily they trust you too. When you treat them humanely, they treat you humanely too. All these years, I've done thousands of abortions now and I never had a lawsuit against me, even though some patients have had complications."

Again like Bennett, Morgentaler soon found abortions overwhelming the rest of his general practice. In early 1969, Morgentaler wrote a letter to all his patients, informing them that he would be specializing in family planning and was terminating his general practice. Such a step, while deemed necessary by Morgentaler, was not an easy one to take. "I felt very regretful, because I got attached to my patients and had developed a long relationship with them – from 1955 to 1969 . . . and some of these people get attached to you. In fact, maybe a dozen insisted on remaining as my patients, and I didn't discourage that too much, so some continued to come. I remember a Ukrainian woman of seventy-five, with high blood pressure, continued to see me another fifteen years. She was a non-Jew but somehow she knew Yiddish songs."

Morgentaler's abortion practice grew rapidly from 1968 till 1970. Though he did not advertise the fact that he performed abortions, word spread quickly, and he received referrals from other doctors in Montreal, and soon, from all over Canada. Similarly, his patients also served as a referral source. He soon came to the attention of the Clergy Consultation Service in the United States and began to receive many patients through this network. When asked to account for the fact that the Montreal police did not raid him in the first two years of his quite visible abortion practice, Morgentaler replied, "The police knew about the damage done by bad abortionists and they didn't particularly care to arrest me because they knew it was a good place, and they had a place where they could send their wives and daughters and mistresses. As long as there were no complaints from anybody, they weren't particularly interested to close down someone providing good service."

In June 1970, Morgentaler's clinic in Montreal was raided, setting off the first of many legal contests between Morgentaler and Canadian prosecutors that would extend over the next twenty years, and indeed which continue to the present day. The circumstances of the first raid involved a tipoff to the FBI by the boyfriend of a woman from the United States who was en route to Canada to receive an abortion from Morgentaler. The FBI in turn alerted the Montreal police, who raided the clinic while the woman in question was in the recovery room. The boyfriend, who was being held on marijuana possession, apparently offered this information in the hope of receiving a lighter sentence.

Various legal skirmishes postponed Morgentaler's first trial until October 1973, and in the period between the raid and the trial, he became even more of a national presence in Canadian abortion politics. In April 1973 (shortly after the *Roe* decision in the United States), he spoke to a large crowd in Toronto of the by-then five thousand abortions he had performed in Montreal with an excellent safety record. Shortly thereafter he invited a television crew into his Montreal clinic and, with the patient's permission, he performed an abortion which was broadcast on a national television network.[10] Morgentaler's motivation was to demonstrate to the Canadian public the safety of clinic-based abortions – and hence the inappropriateness of the 1969 Canadian Abortion Law which permitted only hospital-based abortions.

Morgentaler's first trial, before a French Canadian jury, began in October 1973. He and his attorneys had made a calculated risk that a French Canadian – rather than an English – jury offered the best hope for acquittal. The differences between the refugee physician and his jury were, to be sure, formidable. As Morgentaler put it, "They had nothing in common with me except our common humanity. I was a Jew, I was an atheist, I didn't swear on the Bible [in court], and the foreman of the jury asked the judge about that. . . . I spoke with a European accent, a different French from theirs, I was from a different social class. And the prosecutor made an appeal to this kind of difference. He said, 'Here is a guy who comes to this country, an immigrant, the country treats him well, he graduates from medical school, he has a thriving medical practice, he's a success, and he wants to change our laws.'"

Morgentaler spoke to the jury about his sense of "moral duty" to help those seeking his services. It was also amply clear to this jury that French Canadians had far less access to hospital-based abortion services than did their English-speaking counterparts, as the Catholic hospitals refused to permit abortions. As Morgentaler said, "Obviously these jurors could identify with women who could not get the services and who are obliged to go to back alley butchers and things like that." The jury was further impressed with the testimony of various social service agency representatives that Morgentaler had routinely lowered or waived his fees for low-income women.

After a four-week trial, Morgentaler was acquitted by this jury which in some ways was so different from him. "We proved I was doing it with good motivation. I didn't have evil intentions, I did it with a lot of dexterity, I had a good reputation, the patient had good results. . . . They believed me in spite of what separated us, which was great. It reaffirmed my faith in humanity in a sense."

Immediately after this acquittal, however, the Government of Quebec appealed the jury decision to the Quebec Court of Appeal. This appeal was taken under an until-then never used section of Ca-

nadian law, enacted in 1930, which allows the Court of Appeal to cancel a jury verdict and substitute its own. The Court of Appeal found
Morgentaler guilty and sentenced him to an eighteen-month jail sentence. The Supreme Court of Canada upheld this verdict in March
1975, and Morgentaler immediately began to serve his sentence in a
Montreal jail. Ultimately he was tried twice more before a jury for
the original abortion offense, and each time he was acquitted. After
his third acquittal, which came ten months into his jail sentence, a
newly elected government in Quebec announced that it would no
longer try this case, and furthermore that physicians providing safe
abortions in Quebec would no longer be subject to prosecution. The
strange–and to many, outrageous–nature of Morgentaler's legal
saga, in which the government repeatedly tried him in the face of
three jury acquittals–became a controversy in its own right in Canada among civil libertarians, transcending the abortion issue *per se.*
A former prime minister, John Diefenbaker, introduced a bill which
would no longer allow the Court of Appeals to overturn a jury verdict
of "not guilty"; a new trial would be permissible only in cases of error
of law. Ultimately this bill passed as the Morgentaler Amendment.[11]

Morgentaler's ten months in prison were tumultuous ones. On the
one hand, his self-esteem was intact. "I knew I was there unjustly;
they had overturned my jury acquittal. It was outrageous. I had the
firm conviction that I had done a unique service and should be given
a medal, instead of going to jail!" Yet, faced with the petty humilia-
tions and arbitrariness of prison life–which inevitably brought back
memories of his concentration camp experience–he decided that he
had no choice but to confront prison authorities. "I had to keep my
dignity. . . . In order to get away from the humiliation, I needed to fight
the Administration. There were lots of things to fight about." Morgentaler organized petition drives among prisoners to protest restrictive
visiting policies, advocated for better health care for prisoners, and
served as "father confessor and medical advisor" to many individual
inmates. On one occasion, for instance, he went to the prison kitchen
and asked to speak to the chef. "I told him, 'It isn't good dietetics to
give four eggs one day and none the rest of the week. It is too much
cholesterol. I have some knowledge of dietetics, being a doctor, and I

just want to give you that advice.'" Laughingly, he recalled meeting a fellow inmate years after they were both released and asking, "Tell me, how did you see me in prison? How did I act?" The former prisoner replied, "You walked around as if you owned the place."

Prison authorities, not surprisingly, considered Morgantaler a troublemaker. He was not released after six months, when he had served one third of his sentence, which would have been the norm for prisoners with good behavior. He was put in solitary confinement at one point, until he threatened that he would expose such practices and was released. While in prison, Morgentaler, then fifty-two, suffered a mild heart attack and had to spend part of his sentence in a convalescence hospital.

After his release from prison in 1976, Morgentaler resumed his medical work in Montreal. After a relative respite of several years from politics, and having been able to pay off his considerable legal debts from his earlier campaigns, he decided to launch the "second phase" of his abortion struggle – to extend safe abortion services to other Canadian provinces. In 1983, he opened clinics in Winnipeg and Toronto. Both were promptly raided by the police, again involving Morgentaler in protracted legal battles with provincial governments. In the Toronto case, he and his colleagues were acquitted by a jury, and the government appealed the verdict, which was cancelled by the Court of Appeal. (However, due to the Morgentaler Amendment stemming from the Quebec trials, Morgentaler could not be sent to jail in this case.) Morgentaler in turn appealed to the Canadian Supreme Court, and in January 1988 he achieved the most significant legal victory of his career to date when the Court, in a case bearing his name, declared Canada's abortion law to be invalid.[12]

This 1988 ruling, however, has not resolved all the legal questions governing abortion in Canada. In the absence of any national abortion law to date, struggles over the circumstances under which abortions are to be permitted are being waged in individual provinces, and Morgentaler has been at the center of these battles. Since 1988, he has opened additional clinics in Newfoundland, Nova Scotia, and Alberta, and in each case has been met with varying degrees of legal harassment by provincial authorities (as well as arson attempts,

blockades, and the bombing of one of his clinics by antiabortionists).
In light of this governmental resistance, an especially gratifying victory for Morgentaler has been the turnaround in the province of Quebec, where he started his career of abortion provision. After his release from prison, a newly elected government in the province not
only announced it would not prosecute Morgentaler any longer, but
sought his help in establishing abortion services to be provided in
government-run health clinics in Quebec.

Reflecting on the abortion campaigns of Henry Morgentaler, one
of the most intriguing questions is, simply, why did someone who
had endured so much suffering consciously subject himself to so
much risk? Given the quiet lives chosen by many concentration
camp survivors, it is on the surface puzzling why Morgentaler chose
to engage with the abortion issue after arriving in Canada; why he
continued his abortion struggle after being released from prison,
where he had suffered a heart attack; why today, in his seventies, he
persists in working in clinics that of necessity resemble armed for-
tresses, with demonstrators outside carrying pickets comparing him
to Hitler.

Morgentaler offers several answers to this question. He sees his
long abortion campaign as a powerful emotional connection to his
parents, both murdered when he was still an adolescent. "The fight
for the dignity of humanity was part of my inheritance in a sense." He
further acknowledges that as a result of earlier "crushing" confrontations with authority in the Polish ghetto and in the concentration
camps, he had a psychological need to confront governmental authority, in the face of injustice, in order to become a "full person."
Most compellingly, Morgentaler attributed his abortion activity to
the strong desire – noted in other concentration camp survivors as
well[13] – to lead a life that felt "meaningful."

> There was the desire to do something positive in my life, since this life
> could have been snuffed out. Well, finally I had the chance to do some-
> thing positive . . . something positive in line with counteracting the evil
> that I experienced on my skin, that my family experienced, that my
> people experienced. [I could] try to build a society where children will
> be loved, and desired, and cared for, and therefore would grow up to be

loving, caring persons, who will not build concentration camps, will not rape, maim, or murder. Out of your own courage and your own art that you develop in medicine, you help a person in a terrible predicament, and through the principle that you allow women to have children at a time when they can provide love and affection to them, you build a better society – within the means that are available to you. A society where there will be no more Auschwitzes and no more Dachaus.

CHAPTER FIVE

"I Wanted to Do Something about Abortion": Facilitating Abortions before *Roe*

All the subjects of this book – those I have termed "physicians of conscience" – engaged in various abortion-related activities in the pre-*Roe* era, even if most stopped short of actually performing illegal abortions. Helping patients find qualified providers of abortion was one of the major activities of this larger group, which, admittedly, raises the question of how strictly to define "physicians of conscience." Many U.S. physicians in private practice in the pre-*Roe* era – their exact numbers will never be known – quietly made abortion referrals for selected patients. While the overwhelming majority of these physicians were never detected, let alone prosecuted, for these referrals, such activity nonetheless carried some risk, as occasionally a physician would be arrested for an abortion referral. In 1966, for example, in a highly visible case within the medical community, Leon Belous, a prominent Los Angeles obstetrician/gynecologist, was arrested and convicted for referring a distraught college student to another physician for an abortion.[1] In light of this possibility – however remote – of prosecution, there is a sense in which all the physicians who ever helped patients locate abortion providers might also be considered "conscience physicians." Among the physicians interviewed for this book, however, "facilitating" abortion typically went beyond making referrals. In particular, as it began increasingly to appear that abortion would be legalized in the late 1960s, many of this group took on leadership roles within the medical community, both promoting legalization within the political arena, and preparing the profession for the eventual necessity to provide a new medical service. Their outspokenness on abortion typically led these advocates to encounter the strong distaste for abortion that still existed in much of the medical community, as well as the opposition of a newly emerging antiabortion movement. The main link I find among all the subjects of this book – whatever the degree of their legal risk-taking – was a willingness to be identified with the abortion issue, and hence to subject themselves to the inevitable costs of that visibility.

RELATIONSHIPS WITH ILLEGAL ABORTIONISTS

The extremely negative views of illegal abortionists that many of the physicians interviewed for this book held stemmed from both the longstanding antipathy toward abortionists within medical culture, and, especially, from memorable encounters in hospital emergency rooms with the disastrous consequences of the work of abortionists.

But as these "conscience" physicians' careers progressed, they began to differentiate between "butchers" and competent abortionists (whether lay or physician), both decrying the work of the former and admiring the work of the latter. For example, when Horace Freeman, a physician on the East Coast, first began to do "authorized" hospital abortions in the 1950s, he found the procedure quite challenging (this was in the pre-vacuum suction era): "If I, a trained ob/gyn guy, in an operating room, with lights, with nurses, with a woman under anesthesia ... if I started to do an abortion and my ankles are in blood – how did this guy do it on a kitchen table with a gooseneck lamp and no anesthesia?! I never could figure it out. They knew something I didn't, and of course I never was able to figure out what that was."

The increasing realization, on the part of mainstream physicians, that desperate women would *always* seek out abortions also led to a more sympathetic posture toward illegal practitioners. Indeed, as these physicians made the shift from residency to private practice and started to develop relationships with their patients, they would typically recieve their first request for an abortion – or at the least, for an abortion referral. Thus, while still contemptuous of incompetent abortionists, these physicians simultaneously began to search for reliable abortion providers to whom they could refer their own patients.

Taylor Buckley's "arrangement" with a nurse was typical of the relationships that many doctors established in the pre-*Roe* era. Buckley's roots were in a wealthy and socially prominent family on Philadelphia's Main Line. His medical practice in a large East Coast city, from the 1930s until his retirement in the early 1980s, consisted of a private practice, with patients from social circles similar to his own, as well as considerable public health work. His ambivalence about abortion – or more precisely, about abortionists – was overridden by his sense of obligation to his private patients who needed this service.

On the one hand, Buckley was contemptuous of many illegal abortionists whose ineptitude became evident when their patients appeared in the hospital emergency room. On the other hand, in Buckley's own words,

> Every doctor – let's put it very frankly – who wanted to help people had to
> have an abortionist that he trusted. And I had a nurse out near Lake
> County. She had a very nice place. And an honest kid came in one day
> and said she wanted a checkup for her abortion which she had just had,
> two weeks ago. And I found her in excellent shape. And I said, "Do you
> mind telling me who?" She gave me all the particulars and I called the
> woman. She said, "Why don't you come out and see me?" I went out and
> she had a nice old house – immaculate. She had two or three nurses
> working for her. She had been trained in one of our best hospitals and
> did a precise and clean job.

Buckley referred, in his estimation, about a dozen women a year to this nurse. He offered this referral only to those in his private practice or personal network – not to the "ward patients" whom he saw in the hospital. While acknowledging that such referrals were illegal, and that he was putting himself at some risk by sustaining this relationship with the nurses, he nonetheless stated: "Well, let me tell you this. Every doctor I knew well, who was in my specialty, had someone. Now, it was something you didn't talk about, even with your best friends. But when doctors' families . . . let's say a doctor would come to you and say, 'Look, my daughter ..' well, you had to have some place that you could send people that you wanted to help. . . . They [patients] trusted you and you trusted them. . . . I think anybody is totally heartless who doesn't help out some youngster who is full of anguish over her pregnancy."

In spite of Buckley's evident compassion for women in desperation over unwanted pregnancies and his particular sense of obligation to his colleagues who needed help for family members, it is nonetheless noteworthy that he was scrupulously silent about his arrangement with the nurse. When asked why he was so reluctant to discuss this matter with other physicians, his answer was straightforward: "Honestly, you didn't want a string of these patients coming to you for help. You didn't want to be known as the person who everybody who needed an abortion would come to." Buckley's referral practices thus reinforce the point that there was a broad continuum of abortion facilitators, ranging from those who were willing to undergo minimal risk for a few patients to those whose activities were more far-reaching (and riskier). Though before *Roe* Buckley was an outspoken advocate for legalized abortion (and after *Roe*, established abortion services in several hospitals), his highly selective and discreet referrals placed him at one end of this continuum.

It was common for physicians with patients who could afford it to refer women to practitioners abroad. Mexico and Puerto Rico were major destinations for women from the United States seeking abortions in the years preceding *Roe*. Though the procedure was technically illegal there as well, many clinics apparently operated with impunity. Though women from all over the United States went to Mexico, most who did so were from the West Coast and the Southwest. Tania Meadows, who was in general practice in California in the mid-1960s, recalls a particularly energetic referral source: "There was this huge network going down to Mexico and there were lots of people involved in this, going back and forth to Mexico to check out clinics and doctors, including one man who had a sort of mobile van, and he could connect your telephone call with the clinic in Mexico. He was way ahead of his time in terms of the technology, and he would make a certain amount of money through these referrals, so some people were suspicious of him, but actually he did an extremely good job, and he would go back and forth checking on his Mexican connections."

As Meadows's comments suggest, "quality control" was a particular concern of those – both physician and lay groups – who were making referrals outside the country. As with domestic referrals, the best sources of information for the physicians were the verbal reports and physical condition of returning patients. An added advantage, in the minds of the referring physicians, was that the foreigners to whom they were referring were also physicians. Besides trying to identify those Mexican and Puerto Rican abortion providers who were the most medically adept, a major concern both of those interviewed for this study and others who were making such referrals at the time[2] was the apparently wide variation in ethical standards among the clinics in these countries. Besides significant differences in cost, availability of English speakers to explain the procedure, cleanliness, accessibility, and so on, how the patient could expect to be treated varied enormously. As an extreme example of such concerns, Sheldon Rothstein, who as a New Yorker often made referrals to Puerto Rico, recalled with frustration one doctor who did "technically good work" but who was known to make sexual advances to his patients.

In the other countries in which referrals were common in the pre-*Roe* period – Japan, England, Sweden – abortion was legal, and thus the norms of professional responsibility, i.e., reporting back to the referring physician, could more easily be observed. Charles Swensen, in practice in the Pacific Northwest in the 1960s, developed a very positive working relationship with a physician in Japan: "Well, somewhere along the line, a patient came to see me for a postoperative examination. I was very impressed that she was very normal, she did well, and she confided that she had flown to Japan. Dr. Fukima [not his real name], who I eventually talked to on the phone, though never had a chance to meet personally, obviously was skilled and as time went on he would send letters, he would send little notes with patients indicating what he had done, how things had gone. . . . It was a nice arrangement, but of course it was very expensive."

Similarly, Ed Lever, a physician in the Midwest in the late 1950s and 1960s, got the name of a London physician and was able to maintain a professionally appropriate relationship with him. "I sent a letter with the patient, an open envelope that she could read. A few weeks later I would get a letter from the physician, 'I saw your patient, Mrs. Jones, this is what I found, this is what I did, these are the medications, and please let me know if things don't go well,' and it was very professional."

Of course, foreign referrals were of use only to those who could afford them. While prices varied considerably, several doctors quoted a figure of $1000 charged by Puerto Rican doctors for the operation alone; the Mexican clinics appeared to have charged in the $500 or less range. Abortions in Japan were apparently considerably cheaper, but the airfare was steep. Some women, of course, would do anything possible to get a safe abortion. Rosalind Greene, who practiced in an impoverished New England setting, recalled an operating room nurse "who went to the bank and took out a loan to get to Japan, and she had her operation, and eventually paid off that loan." In the vast majority of cases (with the exception of women who lived in driving distance of the Mexican border), however, the foreign abortions were an option only for the well-off.

Two developments in the immediate pre-*Roe* era made the referral situation considerably easier for abortion-sympathetic physicians: the formation of the Clergy Consultation Service, which started in New York in 1967 and soon spread across the country, and the easing of abortion restrictions in certain key states in the late 1960s and early 1970s. The CCS made both domestic and international referrals. Ed Lever, for example, made contact with the major CCS minister in his city and, though Lever found him somewhat "weird" and a bit of a publicity hound, he nonetheless trusted his judgment on abortion referrals. "He had sent patients to my office who had had abortions and I saw they were all doing very well. And they had been treated with antibiotics . . . so he and I met, we talked, and I started to refer patients to him, telling the patients this is the man who will make some referrals."

Caleb Barrington, in residency in the Midwest in the late 1960s and early 1970s, described how the CCS "streamlined" abortion services. "If you wanted an abortion legally done, one by a physician, you could fly to Japan for the weekend and get back. So . . . the Clergy Counseling Service had a set-up where they had all the paper work, so you could get your visa quickly, get their yellow fever shots, whatever it took to fly into the Orient, and within a week, have all the paper done so they could take three to four days for those who wanted it done legally." (George Jacobs, also in practice in the Midwest in this period, recalls receiving ads at his office about Japanese abortion services: "Ads from Japan, saying, 'Fly your patient to Japan. She'll be met by an English-speaking driver and taken straight to the clinic.'")

Barrington, who became very visible in his community because of his outspoken advocacy of legalized abortion, soon was directly approached by the CCS. The Service asked his help both in getting women approved for therapeutic abortions at his hospital and in providing back-up services to those women the Service was referring to out-of-state abortion facilities.

> They asked me, "Would you check these patients before they go and find out how far along they are, so they don't at sixteen weeks get to New York City, in an outpatient situation, and have a problem." [The free-standing clinics in New York at that time would typically not do an abortion on someone that far along in pregnancy.] Secondly, if they were having a problem, would you check them afterwards so that the patients know that somebody's going to see to it that everything's done properly. . . . Once I took one [CCS patient], suddenly there was a large number there during my noon hour. I would be in the women's hospital, which had a little treatment room just near the door of the hospital, where patients who thought they might be in labor would come to get checked and then be admitted to the hospital. . . . So I said to myself, "This is an ideal place to check somebody to see if they're pregnant or how far along they are," and I would just fill out a little prescription pad, "Patient so and so is so many weeks pregnant by history and exam." . . . So I was spending a lot of my lunch hours checking three to four patients a day sometimes.

When patients returned to Barrington for a postabortion checkup, he closely questioned them on their experience: "I would ask what was done to them. If it sounded shady or had been done without any anesthesia, or you could hear screaming patients in the next room, or it just sounded like a bad situation, I would have them tell CCS. I didn't even know who their CCS counselor was. I didn't know the person that they had seen, in fact they [counselors] would rotate every week, so every clergyman we knew would take their week's stint."

Summarizing his contribution to the efforts of the CCS, Barrington said,

> I was trying to do some kind of quality control. . . . One of the interesting
> things at that time was the number of letters I got from patients. Grate-
> ful letters for having been there for them when they needed somebody,
> because they were of course terrified when they were going – early on
> they were going to Chicago or Detroit for procedures which were done
> behind a sheet, with them not knowing if there was a doctor there or
> not, or what was happening. All the clergy counseling could do was
> ask – was the outcome good or bad? If somebody had a bunch of patients
> come out with bad results, they [CCS counselors] needed to talk to each
> other and say they better not send to that person anymore. . . . I was part
> of the quality control there in that sense.[3]

Frequently the "above-ground" physician took on a more collaborative role with the illegal abortionist he or she had found. Miriam Harkin's activities were particularly interesting in this regard and suggest the lengths to which a sympathetic physician would go, short of actually performing abortions. Harkin was born in the rural Midwest in the 1920s. One of her major childhood memories is overhearing her parents' discussing the traumatic death of Harkin's aunt after an illegal abortion. "She had six kids, twins in diapers. . . . One day my mother said Clara was very sick and she had to go sit with her. She stayed with her the whole night. . . . When she came back, she said she had died, and she described to my dad what it was like before her death, high fever delirium, chewing lips from the pain. It was pretty well known that she had died of an abortion attempt by a well-meaning country doctor."

Another trauma occurred many years later, in the 1960s, when Harkin was in practice as an ob/gyn in a large Midwestern city. As one of the few women in practice in that city at the time, she frequently was approached by patients who wanted abortions. For those whom she felt had a chance to qualify, she would attempt to obtain an abortion through the machinery of her hospital's therapeutic abortion committee. "Around 1967, this woman called, and I said, 'Yes, I will be glad to help you, but first I want you to see Dr. So and So, and do so and so,' and I began to set up appointments. . . . She was home from college for her Christmas vacation. I said, 'Let's get this all lined up.' I didn't realize how desperate she was. . . . I think the route I presented her was just too much to handle . . . I was probably her last hope. Well anyway, I found out later that she just went back to her college and jumped out of her dormitory window. . . . I read about it in the newspaper."

This experience only intensified Harkin's already existing sympathy to her patients' need for abortion, but she felt constrained from performing illegal abortions herself because of her personal situation. "I wanted to do something about abortion, but I was divorced and had four little kids I was supporting and I couldn't afford to have my license jerked."

Through a patient of hers – "a very decent, liberal person" – Harkin came to have contact with "Mickey," a lay abortionist who was the patient's boyfriend. The initial contact occurred when one of Mickey's abortion cases called Harkin. "He had a patient who got into a real jam, but he wasn't the type to run away, so he had his patient call me. She had a very high fever, and said, 'I'm having a miscarriage, I'm very sick' – but I suspected an abortion (we always suspected an abortion in those days) – and when we got face to face, she confided in me, and so I treated her. She came in the hospital with a temperature of 107 and required intensive care. She went back to Mickey, and now he knew that I could be trusted. He knew from the girlfriend that I had compassion, now he knew he had a source of care."

Out of this incident, Harkin and Mickey developed a relationship that lasted several years (but involved only a few face-to-face meetings). Early on, she requested of the lay abortionist that he give her a list of the names of all those on whom he had performed an abortion: "I wanted to see how his patients had done, if I was seeing any of them in the hospital. . . . From the grapevine, I had been hearing good reports about him. I was very reassured after that. The one patient that I referred directly to him gave me a very good report." Harkin's collaborative activities with Mickey consisted of providing emergency care for patients who required it, obtaining antibiotics for him to distribute to his patients, and giving occasional advice over the telephone. Harkin felt that Mickey's technique was essentially a sound one: "He took IUDs, he put them in boiling water so they would straighten out, and, using a sterile technique, he would slide that IUD into the uterus. He gave them terrimicin; I ordered some antibiotics for him wholesale from a supply house. I felt his patients needed to be covered with antibiotics." Summarizing her collaboration with Mickey, Harkin said, "I sort of felt I mopped up after him."

When trying to understand Harkin's willingness to collaborate with such an individual, we might understand her reasoning as a sort of balancing act: on the one hand, she had doubts about him not being an M.D., but they were offset by her firsthand confirmation of his sense of responsibility – that he was "not the type to run away"; similarly her qualms about his not being a physician were offset by her realization that "very few M.D.s at the time had the courage to do what he was doing"; finally, her own guilt at not providing abortions herself was offset by her willingness to collaborate with this provider (and in fact to put herself in some jeopardy by doing so).[4]

Harkin's relationship with Mickey petered out after two years when the Clergy Consultation Service became active in her community and she was able to obtain referrals to *bona fide* physicians, both elsewhere in the United States and in Mexico.

Not all such collaborative relationships between mainstream physicians and providers of illegal abortion worked so well. Sheldon Rothstein, in private practice in New York City in the 1950s and 1960s, was highly sympathetic to women seeking abortions and he sought to help out "decent" abortion providers. In Rothstein's case, such a relationship had been already been modelled for him by the example of his father, also an obstetrician/gynecologist. Though Rothstein's father periodically condemned "abortionists" as "greedy" and unethical, the older physician had a very close working relationship with Robert Spencer, the legendary abortionist based in Pennsylvania from the 1930s through the 1960s. "Spencer was in the medical corps during World War I with Dad and Dad said he was one of the finest young surgeons he had ever met. . . . He really did it because he believed in it. Most criminal abortionists were not of this ilk." Rothstein senior referred many patients to Spencer (as his son also would later do) and occasionally consulted with the Pennsylvania doctor as to the management of patients with complications.

The younger Rothstein for a time agreed to serve as an advisor/ consultant to Dr. Ludwig, a New Jersey pediatrician who performed illegal abortions (and to whom Rothstein occasionally referred patients). After Rothstein was called upon to complete an abortion that Ludwig had bungled, Ludwig increasingly turned to him for help, but Rothstein came to realize that his protege, though well intentioned, was simply too inept medically, and that their professional relationship was a serious mistake.

> He would call me from time to time with a problem. . . . One hot June day, I got a telephone call, "Hello, Dr. Rothstein, this is your friend in New Jersey and I think maybe I got a little bit of a problem." "What's the matter?" "I think maybe I removed a little bit of her small intestine." I said, "Where is the specimen?" and he says, "In the bucket." I said, "Put the specimen in something and send them to see me." So it was one of the few days at that point in my career where I was really busy, and a couple hours went by and it completely jumped out of my head, and I'm going about my business at my office, and the doorbell rang, and everybody was busy as hell, and I opened the door, and there was this liveried chauffeur and [he said] "I'm from Dr. Ludwig in New Jersey." I said, "Where's the patient?" "She's in the car, doc." So I went out with him and there is a seven-passenger caddie with the hood up, and I walk around the hood and I see a middle-aged woman sitting in the back seat. I said to the chauffeur, "Where is the patient?" With a flourish he opens the door and where the jump seats are is this young kid lying on the floor. I took her pulse and it was very rapid but strong and next to her head is a brown paper bag, so once I took her pulse I left her, and took the bag and went back into my office and what was in the paper bag was her small intestine.
>
> I then called the hospital, got a bed in the ICU and got a general sur-

geon and sent them on down. I proceeded to finish my office hours while she was being admitted and while the general surgeon was doing his thing. I then went in and her belly was open from the bowel section; she had to have what was called an end-to-end anastomosis.

What happened was the guy perforated; he thought it was the cord and pulled out – they measured it in the laboratory – eight feet of small bowels. . . . He panicked and blew his cool. He got the eight feet out and you know what he did? He cut it with scissors and then he put it in the bucket and then he called me.

So she's in the hospital. She had a bowel repair, and the general surgeon finished and everybody is telling me to do a hysterectomy on this seventeen-year-old kid from Birmingham, Alabama, no children. I decided no. She had a hole in the top of her uterus; I opened it up and removed the fetus. . . . We sewed up the uterus and I get done with the case, and I'm told the fuzz are looking for me. I haven't done anything illegal. Now I'm not going to go to jail for this guy but on the other hand, I'm not going to blow the whistle on him. That is up to the family. Nobody elected me god.

Well, they [police] were waiting for me at one entrance and I went out the other. The next day the aunt, who was the lady in the back of the limousine, hired a former district attorney. It was her decision to protect the doctor. Well, had the patient died, I would have been implicated. The fuzz came after me and I played dumb and I said, "You have to talk to the patient." The former D.A. said, "You can't talk to the patient, she's too sick." The doctor paid the entire hospital bill, and he also paid me a fee, and he also paid the general surgeon a fee. The patient had a very stormy course but she left the hospital with her reproductive organs and she was okay. . . . What I do want to know, and I always wondered about these many, many years, was whether this kid ever had any children.

Rothstein terminated his relationship with Dr. Ludwig after this incident, but he, like so many others in this study, constantly was on the lookout for reliable abortionists to whom he could refer patients.

HOSPITAL-BASED ACTIVITY IN THE PRE-*ROE* ERA

In the hospitals in which they had staff privileges, these conscience physicians were involved in abortion in two significant ways: they advocated on behalf of patients with their hospital's therapeutic abortion committees, and they performed officially approved abortions.

To recapitulate, although each state's laws gave broad guidelines as to which abortions were legally permitted, the implementation of these laws (including the interpretation of often vague language such as "threat to the health of the mother") were, by the 1960s, in most instances left to the abortion committees – typically consisting of physicians from a variety of fields – that were established in individual hospitals. Hence, the availability of a hospital abortion in a particular place depended not only on the laws of a particular state, but also on the more informal medical and political climate in that region, and even in an individual hospital.

I have already suggested, in chapter 3, that an important component in the development of this group's pro-choice sensibility was their experience, as residents, of viewing the often arbitrary and unfair workings of hospital abortion committees. Although as full-fledged physicians, they had considerably more status and power than they had as residents, still the dealings with the abortion committees could be enormously frustrating. Miriam Harkin described the often frantic procedures she had to go through to get a patient approved:

> Well, to prepare her for the committee, she would write a letter, the spouse would have to write a letter, and then I would quickly have to get consultants. Get her to a psychiatrist. If she had high blood pressure, I could get her through on a medical, but I'd have to call and beg them to see her quickly. I'd put a note in her hand and send her right over. And let's say I would send her to an office, and she wouldn't see my contact, but a colleague who was antiabortion. It required a lot of orchestration to make sure everything went right. The same thing with psychiatrists – if she didn't see the right one, it was trouble. I had to make sure she saw the right one. If she didn't, then she'd come back here and we'd start all over. She'd have to insist to the doctor that she needed his note, right away, right that day, and not have him dictate it for later, the way they usually do. It was just an incredible hassle. And with all those letters in hand, we'd have to go before a scheduled meeting of the committee. And if the committee was not going to meet, we'd have to call each of them by phone.

Although Harkin acknowledged that most of those she brought to the committee were ultimately approved for an abortion, she also admitted to being selective, in order to protect those whom she felt had no chance: "There were people who I would not bring, because I knew they would go through two consultants, bare their souls, and then not get through."

Charles Swensen also reported enormous difficulties dealing with the therapeutic abortion committee in his hospital in the Northwest.

> The committees were not usually made up of obstetricians and gynecologists; they were made up of physicians of other disciplines who seldom, if ever, faced the social issues that people are more comfortable with today. They were people who would say, "Well, we all have bad luck," all those kinds of things, a very self-righteous group, so I went through a couple of things – I remember seeing a woman with exposure to rubella and it was never a clear diagnosis if she had rubella at that time. . . . We didn't have the blood test to clarify just what was going on. We got an opinion from a so-called expert at the university and he couldn't give us a clear answer. She was denied and she went off and received an abortion in Japan.

Even physicians who did not report having been frustrated in dealing with therapeutic abortion committees nonetheless recalled with some distaste the "charades" they underwent on behalf of some patients seeking abortions. Victor Black was working in a hospital in California in the late 1960s when the law passed which permitted abortions on mental health grounds.

> As a result the floodgates were opened. We were ahead of everyone else, especially in our area, and started doing abortions immediately, almost entirely on psychiatric grounds. . . . In historical perspective, this is significant in that we were able to do the abortions, but the type of process the woman had to go through to get it was very demanding. I think we all felt this very keenly, it was a joke, a charade. . . . The patient would call, want an abortion, and we would tell her she had to see two psychiatrists. At first, we had our in-house psychiatrist see them. He became so busy, immediately, that he only had time to do abortion consultations.

He finally told us he didn't have time to see anyone else and that he couldn't do it anymore. . . . We found three or four sympathetic doctors in the area that agreed to see these patients immediately and always agreed that the patient needed an abortion. All had the same diagnosis: "situational anxiety." These were all normal women, in my opinion, with no psychiatric problems. But these were the hoops they had to go through.

Horace Freeman, in practice in New England in the late 1960s, recalled the addition of the mental health clause as a very positive step, as most of those seeking abortions did not have physical indications. "Once you'd got the word 'mental' in there, you were home free." At the same time, Freeman saw a negative side to this new policy: "The patient had to go through the terrible charade of going to a psychiatrist and getting a $50 letter which was sent to me which said that she would commit suicide or some drastic step. . . . This was a demeaning experience. What if this woman at some future date ever wanted to apply for a job, or ever wanted to get credit cards and they looked up her hospital records – they would find that she was going to commit suicide, which of course was phony."

The mental health clauses thus made for a sometimes awkward situation between referring physician and collaborating psychiatrist. On the one hand, the former were dependent on the latter to obtain abortions for patients; on the other, a certain degree of contempt inevitably arose on the part of some referring physicians, as they saw psychiatrists cynically profiting from the clause. Sheldon Rothstein described his relationship with consulting psychiatrists in the late 1960s in these terms: "I would refer patients for psychiatric consultation back in 1969 and it was $75 for a very short interview, and I had several psychiatrists in my stable, so to speak, and one of them made up a form letter. 'This blank-year-old blank-for-race female whose last menstrual period was blank is pregnant and the pregnancy constitutes a threat to her life because blank.' They would fill in three or four different things. It was basically a form letter. I said to my stable of guys, "You don't take Medicaid patients, you don't get my private referrals." And they did, but they didn't want to. They would take my private patients at $75 and $50 for ten minutes, fifteen minutes."[5]

One obvious solution to the problem of dealing with recalcitrant or arbitrary therapeutic abortion committees was for abortion-sympathetic physicians to get themselves appointed to these committees. Irving Goodman recalled a particularly frustrating case in which a patient of his had been turned down by the hospital's committee. "Myself and one of my other colleagues, we went to the department chair to complain, and as far as he was concerned, he didn't care. I said, 'Come on, Larry, let's get this over with.' He says, 'I have nothing to do with it, the committee does.' And I looked at him and said, "Next year the committee is up for reappointment. Are you going to appoint me on the committee or are you going to reappoint him [an antiabortion colleague]'? He looked at me and said, 'Okay.' So I joined the committee. As soon as the committee was changed, by one person willing to appoint the right people, the issue [of obtaining approved abortions] was moot in our organization."

Miriam Harkin ultimately managed to get herself appointed head of the therapeutic abortion committee in her hospital. But even with sympathetic colleagues on her committee, Harkin felt constrained from approving abortions for all who sought them; she was well aware that without some appearance of selectivity, her committee's decisions might be overridden. She and her colleagues therefore colluded on a "triage" plan – "sometimes it boiled down to whether she could afford the airfare to get to a legal abortion in another state. We tried to save the slots here for those we knew could not." As Harkin pointed out, even an approved patient often faced emotional difficulties in the hospital. "Even those we got through the committee, the nurses were absolutely cruel. I can remember one woman who was forty, had hypertension – we got two consultants to say an abortion was necessary to save her life, we went through all these time-consuming procedures. Finally she got the abortion." It so happened she had twin fetuses, and it was on the hospital chart. When the nurses saw her chart, they took her down to the nursery, and showed her twins that had just been born. And this was in a hospital where the nurses were wonderful nurses, caring nurses – the hospital where I did my practice, and the nurses were my friends!"

Nearly all of those interviewed for this study also report having performed hospital-approved abortions themselves in the pre-*Roe*

era. In some instances – depending on the political climate both lo-
cally and within the hospital itself, as well as of course the indication
for the abortion – these operations were nonremarkable occurrences.
That is, the patient's request would be duly certified by the therapeutic abortion committee and the doctor would proceed with the operation. In other instances, however, performing an abortion – even an
"approved" one – was a far more complex affair, since physicians performing committee-approved abortions could never be entirely sure
that there would not be oversight from external legal authorities.
Thus, such hospital-approved abortions in this pre-*Roe* period have
been termed by some as "gray area" abortions, because of the chronic
uncertainty of their legality. Two participants spoke of having infor-
mally asked district attorneys about the possibility of being prosecuted for doing hospital abortions. Rosalind Greene, on a medical
school faculty in New England, began to participate in community-
based forums on abortion in the mid-1960s. Through this work, she
became acquainted with Michael Cannon (not his real name), the
county district attorney, later to become a well-known congressman.

> One night Mike and I were on a panel at one of the Protestant churches,
> discussing abortion, and he said at that time he felt convinced that free-
> dom of choice about abortion was guaranteed under the Constitution,
> and the Supreme Court would uphold it, and as we were going out, we
> came down the church steps together, he and I. We never knew each
> other real well, but we knew each other from that kind of association,
> and I said something about trying to set up to do [hospital-based] abor-
> tions, and he looked at me and said, "Rosalind, I would never prosecute
> you for doing abortions." He was the district attorney of that county and
> that was very helpful to know. I didn't particularly want to go to jail, and
> a very different district attorney could have made things difficult.

Greene shortly thereafter became involved in the establishment
of an abortion service at her university's hospital. As in other clinics
at the hospital, Greene and the other physician performing abortions
did so for fees that were to be turned over to her department. This policy was especially reassuring to Greene, given the controversy over
abortion in the community. "We never profited individually from

them.... I liked the fact that I could look anyone in the eye, and say, 'You know, this is not going into my pocket.'"

Ed Lever, in practice in a community that was particularly torn over the abortion issue, felt he was putting himself in legal jeopardy even while performing "approved" abortions. A particularly memorable case was a patient of his, whom he had delivered twice, who was pregnant with a complication that was serious but not life-threatening. Moreover, the patient, though upset and clearly wanting an abortion, was not "suicidal." Lever was concerned that even if he got her through his hospital committee, some zealous abortion foe – either within the hospital or without – would attempt to make trouble.

> I called up the county attorney, who I knew personally from my involvement in the local Democratic party, Bob Cramer [not his real name], who is now a [state] Supreme Court justice. I said, "Bob, I got a problem. I want to do an abortion openly, but it's going to be sort of 'illegal,'" and he said, "I don't give a damn." I said, "Are you saying to me, even if you found out about it, you would not prosecute me?" He said, "I can't tell you publicly... but go ahead and do it." I did do it, and it was done through the therapeutic abortion clinic. I still felt terribly uneasy. I am a person who doesn't mind taking risks in terms of civil disobedience. I ended up in jail [for participation in the civil rights movement] and it didn't particularly bother me, but if my professional life and my license were going to be taken away, that was a different story.

Obviously, then, the existence of machinery that permitted therapeutic abortions in the pre-*Roe* era did not imply that most physicians felt secure using such machinery indiscriminately. This group as a whole was quite selective about which cases they brought to committees and were careful not to be seen to be performing too many hospital abortions. Howard Wellstone's actions typified the practices of some of those interviewed – he performed a mixture of both illegal (out of hospital) and hospital-approved abortions – and in both cases, proceeded very cautiously so as to avoid a reputation that would inevitably bring him a stream of abortion-seeking patients. He maintained an active referral list for women whose abortions he did not choose to perform himself. One case that did move him to seek a committee-approved abortion occurred in the 1950s. "I remember particularly, a classmate of one of my kids in junior high school. And her father was a doctor and they referred this kid to me. It was perfectly apparent that one does not allow a thirteen-year-old kid to carry a pregnancy just because she had been doing a little experimenting. So I referred her to a psychiatrist, who wrote a note, and I think he did feel it would be too traumatic. And I did a D. & C. on her without any trouble."

For younger doctors contemplating performing abortions under the committee system, the example of more senior colleagues could be extremely important. Morris Fischer represents such a case. Fischer came from an orthodox Jewish background and initially had been opposed to abortion on moral grounds. His exposure, as an obstetrical resident, to women suffering from the effects of illegal abortion converted him to a pro-choice position, and this experience moreover was decisive in distancing him from his orthodox religious views. "I began to read, to study. I began to feel that orthodox Judaism was lacking in compassion – that all orthodox religions were lacking in compassion. I felt that one of the qualifications of a good physician, a good health care professional, was not just to know what the dosage of a pill was, or what shot to give, but to be compassionate, and to realize that this woman with the problem needs help and empathy."

But in spite of his change of heart about abortion, Fischer nonetheless felt uneasy, in the early 1960s, when his department chair at a fairly small hospital asked him to set up a therapeutic abortion committee and to provide the abortions that the committee endorsed. Fischer acknowledges that he was apprehensive in part because he was concerned about a loss of status, reflecting the enduring distaste within the medical world for the "abortionist." "There were a couple of doctors around who were doing [illegal] abortions, and were doing lots of them, and they were looked down upon as 'abortion mill' people, so I didn't want to be like them." But his hesitation also stemmed from fears about possible prosecution – "it was before *Roe v. Wade*; they were really still illegal, I thought."

But then the newspapers in his large East Coast city revealed that doctors at an acclaimed university medical center (where Fischer had been a resident) had been doing hundreds of abortions for patients diagnosed with rubella. This revelation about his former mentors was pleasantly astonishing to Fischer and spurred him to establish an abortion service at his own hospital. "I read about the doctors at University Hospital! So Cohen was doing them! Orloff was doing them! Bauer was doing them! [not their real names] So these guys were doing them and these are great guys, who I have a great deal of love and respect for. These are the people at whose feet I sat and learned, and therefore what they were doing made me feel good, because if they could do it, little old me could do it. . . . That's when I started [abortion work]. . . . It gave me a sense of safety and security that they were doing it. . . . I had been scared that someday I would get called into a courtroom and I would have trouble defending myself."

ADVOCACY WORK

This group of physicians also participated in a range of activities that can be considered together under the heading of "advocacy work" for safe and legal abortion: lobbying state legislatures to liberalize state abortion laws; taking part in community forums about abortion; participating in educational sessions to inform fellow physicians about abortion techniques; and, perhaps most significant, in the years immediately before *Roe* when the legalization of abortion began to appear inevitable, working within medical societies and individual hospitals to design standards for the forthcoming massive expansion of abortion services. For many of these respondents, these advocacy activities not only marked their first foray into the political arena, it also gave them their first taste of the antiabortion movement that would become such a factor in the lives of abortion providers in the years ahead.

George Jacobs was in practice in the Midwest in the early 1970s and very active in his local medical society. Observing the liberalization of abortion laws in neighboring states, he attempted a similar move in his own state.

I tried to organize some activity through the local gynecological society to see if we could have some luck in changing the law, and I met with total defeat there. . . . I remember going down to the State House in the capital with a group of physicians, a really good bunch of physicians. One black obstetrician, who was pro-choice, had a seriously retarded child. He had seen so much havoc wrought from criminal abortion on his own population. I thought we had a pretty persuasive case. When we got down there to testify, they had moved the hearing from the usual hearing room to the rotunda of the House of Representatives because it was the largest hearing they'd ever had at the state house. There were protestors on both sides, and my physician colleagues said, "What the hell have you gotten us into?!" That was our first experience that this was going to be such a polarized, bitter struggle . . . with people carrying fetuses and throwing blood at us and that sort of thing. There were a lot of people that didn't want to put up with that and I can understand that.

Ed Lever, at around the same time, was approached by a group of women health activists in his Midwestern city to enlist him in a campaign to liberalize abortion laws. He was initially approached because of his reputation for involvement in political causes. "I had gotten arrested as a physician working for the Medical Committee for Human Rights. . . . I was always in the newspaper so people knew I was a liberal person. . . . I was well known for my liberal views on the race issue. And because of that liberal view I had a lot of indigent black women on AFDC in my practice."

Lever and his associates politicked both at the state legislature and in his local medical society–in each case, without initial success.

We began agitating at the legislature level. Each year we would go to the legislature and we would find somebody to introduce what was then the American Law Institute proposal for changing the law. It would be solidly defeated. This is an ultraconservative Midwest state. . . . About 1966 or 1967 I was made the program chairman of the state gynecological society, so I arranged for a whole day's conference on abortion and I got the the guy who would later become governor of Colorado, Richard Lamm, who was already a known agitator on abortion, to come here and be the keynote speaker.[6] Well, all hell broke loose in the newspapers. I remember being called on the floor of the state obstetrical/gynecological society a "killer of babies," which didn't particularly bother me because I did have some support.

Charles Swensen, in practice in the Pacific Northwest in 1969, immersed himself in efforts to liberalize his state's abortion law. He was motivated to do so by his sense of the precarious legal status of physicians like himself who were performing hospital-based abortions under the aegis of the therapeutic abortion committees. "We didn't know what kind of risk we were taking. It was unknown at that time. . . . In theory if someone were to press charges, we could be indicted for a criminal act, as could the patient. Our state law was clear that abortion was not allowed. In 1969 there was a statewide movement through an organization called "Citizens for Abortion Reform" that put together a referendum . . . that eventually came to the ballot in November 1970." Swensen lobbied within his state medical society for support of this measure but also did a great deal of public speaking, both on television and in public forums. "One time I found myself debating of all places in the basement of a Catholic Church on a Sunday evening. . . . What came out of it was an interesting experience because for the first time I became aware that the people who were going to win the abortion battle for us were our opponents, and the reason they were going to win it for us is because they were so rigid in their thinking. . . . One of my opponents reached down under the table during the debate and pulled out a fetus in a jar. It polarized the audience to my side of the thing." The referendum did pass, and abortions through the first sixteen weeks of pregnancy became considerably easier to obtain in Swensen's state.

Learning about abortion techniques and disseminating this information to the larger medical community was another major advocacy effort of this group. The pre-*Roe* medical community in the United States was marked not only by widely varying laws and informal understandings of when legal abortions were to be performed, but also by considerable variation in individual physicians' knowledge of abortion practice. Such variations were partly a function of geographical region – obviously those sympathetic to abortion who practiced in liberalized environments were in a better position to learn the latest techniques – but they also reflected the efforts individuals made to train themselves, often against the odds. Ron Ehrlich, who was finishing a residency in ob/gyn in the late 1960s, on the East Coast, spoke quite candidly of the unavoidable haphazardness of his early experience doing saline abortions, a technique then commonly used for second trimester abortions. When asked about his training in this method, Ehrlich answered wryly: "My 'training' wasn't 'training.' I *did* saline abortions. I did them in a self-taught manner, and we did them in a very primitive way. We did what we thought was the way to do them.... What we did then we would not do today ... because we would pick up scattered information from all over the country. And most of what we did, we learned on our own; there was no one to ask."

Ehrlich went on to relate the rather unusual circumstances of his board examination in obstetrics/gynecology in 1969, when the examiners began to question him about saline abortions, and it soon became clear that they were doing so not to "test" Ehrlich, but rather to broaden their own knowledge. "The examiners were asking, 'Well, what do you do next, and how do you do this, and what did you use, and how much did you put in,' and so on.... So there wasn't that much information out there then."

Ehrlich's experiences notwithstanding, there were numerous instances, in the years leading up to *Roe*, of pro-choice physicians more successfully preparing their colleagues for what was seen as the inevitable day of legalized abortion. In chapter 2, I have already discussed two especially influential international conferences on abortion held in the United States, one sponsored by Planned Parenthood in 1955, and the other by the Association for the Study of Abortion in 1968. Beyond such major gatherings, the experiences of the interviewees in this study suggest that in the years immediately before *Roe*, a national network of medical abortion activists was beginning to coalesce, with crucial encounters taking place at international meetings as well as in hospital corridors. The experiences of Barry Messinger, a pivotal figure in the promotion of legal abortion within the medical profession around the time of *Roe*, illustrate the many levels at which information on abortion was obtained and disseminated.

Messinger, in the 1960s, was a professor of obstetrics and gynecology at a prominent medical center on the West Coast. He was first directly introduced to the vacuum suction technique by a visiting Israeli colleague. Like virtually all others in this study who had formerly done abortions using only the D. & C. method, Messinger was very impressed with the greater ease and safety of the suction method. As his Israeli friend told him, "Sure you can do abortion this way, we've done it, but you need to find a source of vacuum pumps." Thus, Messinger approached an acquaintance who was a medical engineer to see if the vacuum pumps could be easily produced: "This fellow George was a great engineer, very imaginative, very entrepreneurial guy. And he said, 'Sure, they're easy to make.'" Messinger and a colleague ultimately made their own training film showing the use of the vacuum aspiration method, which was distributed by the Lalor Foundation, the distributor of an earlier film on this method made by a British physician, Dorothea Kerslake.

Messinger was also instrumental in popularizing another important innovation of that period, the Karman cannula. Harvey Karman, a psychologist from California, was an illegal abortionist who gained considerable respect from many mainstream physicians for his allegedly brilliant adaptations of the standard equipment used in abortions. The Karman cannula, made from soft plastic, made early abortions both safer (because it reduced the likelihood of perforation) and less painful.

Demonstrating once again that links between medically respected illegal abortionists and mainstream physicians were common in the pre-*Roe* period, Karman was a frequent participant at medical meetings on abortions, and it was at one such event that Messinger first encountered him.

It was around 1967, and [Karman] came to the city one Saturday afternoon and demonstrated it [cannula] on a patient... and I got invited. And I knew it was truly terrific. Harvey gave me one of those things. I said, "Do you mind if I take one?" He said, "No, here." I said, "Have you ever had any problem with this? Any difficulties or complications?" And he said, "No, I've never had any problem at all." And I discounted that immediately because no matter what you do, even cross the street, you can have a problem sometimes. But I took this thing. And by that time, George [medical engineer] was in the business of making vacuum pumps, with aspirators that were large and stiff. And I said, "George, this is a good thing." And he knew it too. And so he began to manufacture them in the millions. . . . George distributed it around the world.

With the liberalization of his state's abortion law in 1967, Messinger and his associates began to perform many early abortions in his office, within the hospital complex. He and a colleague flew to New York to report on their work shortly before that state liberalized its law. Their major agenda was to convince their New York colleagues of the feasibility of outpatient abortion.

We went to a meeting of the Planned Parenthood doctors . . . and we presented a paper on early abortions . . . and Alan Guttmacher was around, and he predicted there would be . . . outpatient facilities that provided abortion . . . and what we did was to say, well, our office was in the hospital, but we didn't do them in any kind of hospital surroundings, we did them in my office surroundings. At that juncture, we had data suggesting that you could do them in an office and there would be no problem. And we were abiding by the letter of the state law, in the sense that it was in the hospital. . . . I think it [the safety of outpatient abortions] impressed them. Nobody said, "Oh, my god, you can't do that." We clearly had the data and we just got up there and said, "This is the way we did it." There wasn't any disbelief in the crowd. This was very important in New York because I think their law was just about to unfold. . . . So it meant a lot to them in terms of how they were going to gear up.

Alan Guttmacher's prediction, recollected by Messinger, that abortions would someday be offered in outpatient facilities proved to be correct. In July 1970, the repeal of New York state's abortion law took effect, making abortion legal. In response to this development, the Clergy Consultation Service opened one of the first freestanding abortion clinics in the United States, the Center for Reproductive and Sexual Health (also known as "Women's Services"). The first director of the Center was Hale Harvey, a physician from Louisiana to whom the CCS had very successfully referred many patients for illegal abortions. Other such facilities soon opened in New York and shortly thereafter in Washington, D.C.

The CCS had several reasons for opening such a clinic. First, the Service's track record in abortion referral – one hundred thousand referrals to doctors' offices over a three-year period without a fatality – had persuaded the clergy and their medical advisors of the safety of nonhospital abortions.[7] Second, based on its experiences with a wide range of illegal providers, the CCS feared the possibility of economic exploitation of women by some of the providers who would go into business to meet the huge demand that would follow the New York repeal.[8] Third, again based on the widely varying experiences of women for whom the CCS had made referrals, the organization's leaders had become convinced of the importance of the non-medical aspects of the "abortion experience" – the necessity of clearly explaining the procedure, of offering the patient counseling about her feelings about the abortion, of having supportive staff. Thus, Women's Services was established as a nonprofit facility, with the basic cost of an abortion set at $200, but a sliding scale established for those who could not afford the fee, and a principle that no one should be turned away for lack of money. Women's Services also pioneered the role of the "abortion counselor," a feature that was to become commonplace in many of the freestanding clinics established in that era. The abortion counselor was typically a person without medical training – who often herself had had an abortion, either legal or illegal – whose role it was to counsel the patient before the procedure, accompany her throughout the abortion itself, and also "advocate" for patients in general. Such advocacy, in this early stage of the freestanding clinic, meant giving clinic managers feedback from the patients about various aspects of clinic protocol, including the highly sensitive issue of individual doctors' techniques.[9]

The incorporation of the lay abortion counselor into the freestanding clinic during this formative period of abortion services highlights the uneasy alliance that existed then between the women's health movement and the first generation of physicians to provide legal abortion, including a number of those interviewed for this study. Though both groups were obviously joined in their fierce commitment to achieving legal abortion, they were also divided on occasion by issues of both tactics and substance. The actions of the

most militant factions of the feminist health movement (as mentioned in chapter 2) who, during the tumultuous days of the late 1960s
and early 1970s picketed the AMA convention and disrupted a number of state hearings on abortion reform, embarrassed and dismayed
some abortion-sympathetic physicians. From the latter's perspective, the tainting of the abortion rights cause with the extremism of
"women's libbers" made it that much harder to convince both their
(mostly male) dubious colleagues within the medical profession and
(mostly male) politicians within state legislatures of the necessity for
abortion reform.

But perhaps the most difficult aspect of the relationship between
the two allies occurred at the clinic itself. Not surprisingly, it was
hard for many physicians to accept the nonhierarchical ethos of
many of the early clinics, in which many major decisions were made
by consensus, after long hours of staff meetings. The physicians who
worked in these early abortion facilities were usually older than the
lay counselors, who were typically in their twenties, and, for the most
part, the former were not as steeped in the "movement" culture of
that period, in which lengthy meetings about many issues, including
"interpersonal dynamics" within the clinic, were routine. Most significantly, though, the participating physicians had trouble with the
implicit–sometimes, explicit–challenge, posed by the "team" approach of the clinic, to their profession's historic claims to dominance in medical settings. Here we can recall Jane Hodgson's difficulty adjusting to the organizational structure of the Preterm clinic
in Washington, after years of running her own private practice in
Minneapolis: "I was not accustomed to counselors participating in
medical decisions. It was a team approach that was entirely new
to me and not easy, I might add." Daniel Fieldstone, who also had
experience as medical director of one of the first freestanding abortion clinics, was less measured in his recollections of counselor-
physician relations in that period. He remembered a "confronta-
tional" atmosphere in which it was "them – the counselors and the
patients – against us." Speaking of his periodic staff meetings with
counselors, Fieldstone recalled, "I would sit there and spin the shit off
that was being thrown at me, as the emblematic doctor/male/what-

ever. They were angry. You can't believe how angry these people were." Significantly, however, Fieldstone acknowledged that the lay counselors were a crucial source of information about the newly developing field of clinic-based abortions.

> It was a learning time. We were learning from them. It was more confrontational and less collegial than I would have liked. But we were learning about how women needed to prepare for abortions . . . and how abortions should be done, what the qualities were [of a good abortion provider], how they should be done, if someone could really do an abortion well, and others who couldn't. . . . In truth, it was very useful for educating physicians. Some of them were not waiting for the paracervical block [a newly developed technique of local anesthetic] to work. Some of them didn't know how to do a paracervical block. And there were some people who were technically very able but were never able to deal with it. So it was a very rewarding and constructive time. It made you think about lots of things that we were doing to women, and with women, that had never been thought of.[10]

These newly founded freestanding clinics in New York, as well as those established as outpatient facilities in hospitals, very quickly had to respond to an unprecedented number of women seeking abortions. "Our dam burst," as Fieldstone put it. In the first year after repeal, some two hundred thousand women obtained abortions in New York, the majority of them from out of town. Thus, a medical system that had relatively limited experience in delivering abortions was suddenly faced with the task of organizing services for thousands of patients, most of whom would be leaving New York on the day of their procedure.

In Fieldstone's view, the preparatory steps that some within the medical community had taken earlier proved crucial to preventing what could have been a public health emergency. Speaking of the introduction of the suction machine at the ASA meeting in 1968, and the subsequent distribution of these machines to selected medical centers by the Lalor Foundation, Fieldstone said, "That contribution was extraordinarily vital. Because it meant that x number of centers were using and had used, and were training people in vacuum curettage

... and there's a pool of people that were ready when 1970 came around in New York. When we put the program in [elective abortion] in our hospital, there was a vacuum program ready to go.... They [suction abortions] made it more palatable, certainly made it a lot less bloody and a lot simpler."

Similarly, Fieldstone pointed to a second technological break-through in abortions that occurred just before legalization in New York – the development of the paracervical block, a method of using local anesthetic to block pain from cervical dilation.[11] This innovation, in Fieldstone's words, "enabled you to do abortions under local anesthetic . . . and as a derivative of that, it enabled you to do it in a freestanding setting, without anesthesiology, and without a formal operating room." By 1972, Fieldstone reported, the paracervical block was in widespread use in many of the freestanding clinics that had opened in New York.

In 1970, Judith Harmon had just completed a year of internship, during which she had become involved with a group of progressive medical students and doctors, the Medical Committee for Human Rights. While in medical school, she had also worked as a volunteer counselor for the Clergy Consultation Service, both explaining the procedure to the often "terrified young woman and her terrified aunt," and also transporting the abortion patient to her appointment. These experiences spurred her to take a year off before furthering her medical training and to accept a position on the medical staff of Women's Services. Her memories of the earliest days of the clinic are of the inevitable chaos brought about by such an abrupt and enor-mous demand for abortions:

> The clinic was just inundated. There were lines of patients around the
> block every single morning we opened. From 7:00 A.M. to 11:00 P.M., we
> did two eight-hour shifts of all the staff and personnel. Usually one hun-
> dred or more people a day. Seven days a week. And the other remarkable
> thing about this clinic. They had come to New York of course with very
> little notice. The law changed, bingo, overnight, and there wasn't any
> time to plan. One of the things New York does not have is building space
> where you could just set up a clinic instantly, and what Hale did to start
> the clinic was go to one of the "for rent by the hour" medical office build-
> ings which are fairly common in New York. . . . They [the offices] are

kind of generic, a desk, an exam table, and that's it. Of course to run a clinic of that size, we needed a fairly large amount of space, and they did not have space with that size, so we had this large clinic, but it wasn't in the same room during all hours of the day. We had a big board that told us which hours we could use which rooms. . . . We did fortunately have one little central area that we could have all the time, and that's where we put our recovery area and kept our medications and things like that.

Harmon recalled the variety of fellow physicians who performed abortions during the first months of the clinic's operation. Some had extensive experience, having done illegal abortions. "Who knew how to do an abortion?! Hale hired his buddies from all over the country to work in the clinic." One of Harmon's colleagues is of particular interest because his case foreshadows the problems of legitimacy that legal abortion would have in the decades to come. "I can remember one of the very first regular doctors here. . . . This was a guy who was on the faculty of Columbia [Medical School]. . . . He used a fake name when he worked at the clinic. He needed the money because he had a kid in college. He was afraid that if anyone found out he was working at the clinic, then he would be in trouble with the faculty. He didn't know how to do abortions, so I taught him, and he worked, using his fake name." The fear expressed by Harmon's co-worker was probably well founded. Lawrence Lader, a key abortion rights activist of this period and one of the original founders of the pro-choice group NARAL, attempted to establish a freestanding clinic in Washington, D.C., in early 1970, shortly after a landmark ruling by Judge Gesell of the First District Court which declared Washington's antiabortion statute unconstitutional, and hence opened the door to legal abortion in the District. Lader and his colleagues at NARAL were unable to proceed with their plans because of their inability to secure the cooperation of any area physicians who, in Lader's words, "were willing to stand up against the medical hierarchy. . . . The pressures against a physician were too intense. Anyone who cooperated with us could lose his hospital privileges."[12] (A year later, however, an outpatient abortion clinic opened at Washington Hospital Center, and the freestanding Preterm clinic also was established.)

In spite of the atmosphere of confusion that Harmon remembers from the New York clinic's first months, in fact the safety record of this clinic, and of similar facilities, was exemplary. During its first thirteen months of operation, over twenty-six thousand abortions were performed at the Center for Reproduction and Sexual Health, without a death. A highly regarded study by the biostatisticians Christopher Tietze and Sarah Lewit surveyed some seventy-two thousand abortions performed in the year starting July 1, 1970, and definitively established the safety of abortions in freestanding clinics. The study found that the complication rates were *lower* for non-hospital clinics than for hospitals, and also were lower for hospital outpatient cases than for hospital inpatients.[13]

When the first abortion clinics opened in New York, they not only became a source of referrals for physicians in other states, but also a training site, as Eugene Fox's experience illustrates. Fox was in practice in the South in the early 1970s, and became involved with a feminist health group that was making referrals to New York.

> They wanted me to see patients for them. I told them I was uncomfortable sending patients to New York until they had been seen by somebody, whether they were healthy, that sort of thing. And there should be somebody here to see them when they came back. And the other thing, somebody ought to go up there and see what was going on. Who are we sending these people to? Some of these places were terrible. They were just back alley shops that opened their doors. . . . I went up and toured a bunch of those places and looked at them and finally settled on some. At the same time, the ones I settled on, I spent some time there, and learned some techniques myself. . . . I had never used the suction method before.

As the legalization of abortion began to appear increasingly imminent in various states, other interviewees took leadership roles in their communities to prepare for this momentous change. The recollections of Charles Swensen in the Pacific Northwest, and Bob Phillips on the East Coast of this period are illustrative of the dilemmas that sympathetic physicians faced with the coming of legal abortion. Both of these men worried about a too abrupt transition without proper planning. Their key concerns went beyond safety *per se* and reflected their awareness of the controversial history of abortion –

and thus the special burden on abortion providers to proceed with extreme care. Phillips spoke about his caution when he opened one of the first hospital-based abortion clinics in his city.

> When we opened our clinic we would not do the patient the day she was counseled. She had to come back. Because I never wanted to face a patient coming and saying, "You shouldn't have done me." We made it a two-day procedure.[14] Meantime, there's several groups [interested in abortion], we went together to see the head of City Council, to set up standards to see that it didn't turn into a sleaze operation. I could see that coming. . . . Every Tom, Dick, and Harry setting up an abortion clinic and making a million dollars and turning women out like M & M's, as pieces of meat. . . . So, we got the city behind us. We had a large group of people meeting, lawyers, social workers, physicians . . . fifteen or twenty people. We had many ongoing meetings. We set up a set of standards finally.

Charles Swensen, whose efforts to get a liberalized abortion law passed in his state were discussed above, abruptly found himself having to deal with the consequences of his victory. "On November 3 the vote came through, and the law went into effect on December 3 . . . so we had a window there of about a month to reflect on what had happened, and while we were sitting casually with the state attorney general, who was now going to come to grips with this law, we started talking about quality of care, and he said, 'I'm sorry, gentlemen, there's nothing in the law that says the state will play any role in the quality of care.' I said, 'You've got to be kidding.' He said, 'All we can do is to inspect the facilities to make sure they have toilets, enough light, sanitary conditions, and so on.' "

When asked specifically what he had been afraid of, Swensen replied, "First of all, nobody knew how to do an abortion, nobody had been trained. I suddenly said to myself, 'Jiminy Christmas, are we going to have a problem on our hands in a few weeks!' I was on the medical committee [of his local Planned Parenthood affiliate]. I went to them and explained the situation and in a very brief period of time, our committee made the recommendation that we as a committee would be a clearinghouse for physicians who would have to have us at Planned Parenthood refer patients to them for abortions. What that clearinghouse would do, we would physically visit their facilities, we would physically watch them perform an abortion and check their credentials." Swensen's anxiety about the quality of care in his state of course has to be understood in the context of the pre-*Roe* era, when the training and skill among abortion providers – both legal and illegal – varied enormously. The prominence given by the press to the occasional abortion-related death or injury before legalization was very much in Swensen's mind as he contemplated a future of widespread abortion services. "What I realized was that the first accident would be the toughest to defend, and the longer we could put off the first accident, the first death, the first perforation, the first infection, and get more experience and credibility under our belt, the better off we were going to be."

As yet another indication of the very delicate deliberations surrounding the legalization of abortion in Swensen's state, he reported on an unusual step taken by his state's medical society. "The state medical association made the decision that we had to be aware of quality assurance, and on that basis they did not want physicians to become entrepreneurs around abortion. . . . For the first time in the history of the state, and I think the only time, the medical society went on record as recommending a fee, and the fee for abortion was not to exceed the cost of a diagnostic D. & C. In reality what happened was the fees fell below that, and I have never met anyone from any other state in the Union where the cost of abortion was as cheap as [this state] then, nor is there any state in the Union where the fee is cheaper than it is today."

A LIGHT AT THE END OF THE TUNNEL?

The decade leading up to *Roe* was a tumultuous one for abortion-sympathetic physicians. On the one hand, there was the familiar frustration that, in spite of the many efforts made by this group, only a small number of the women seeking abortions could be helped. The difficulty of finding reliable abortion providers, the fear of detection if too many referrals were made, and the conservatism of colleagues on hospital therapeutic abortion committees all were powerful constraints on those attempting to help.

But by the late 1960s and early 1970s, things began to change. A vibrant abortion rights movement had emerged, at both the national and local levels. Many of the physicians who joined these efforts experienced for the first time the complexity of abortion politics beyond the medical community, as they encountered the sometimes uncomfortable support of the more radical wing of the women's health movement and the bitter opposition of the antiabortion movement.

Simultaneous with these political developments, abortion practice changed as well. By 1967, certain states such as California had greatly liberalized their abortion laws, and by the early 1970s, New York and Washington, D.C. had become sites of massive abortion provision. At least for those patients with the resources to travel, now physicians in all regions had reliable places to send them. For these physicians, much of whose careers had been spent seeing the tragedies of illegal abortion, this new availability of legal abortion was – as one participant in this study put it– "a breath of fresh air." Another participant, just starting her second year of residency in New York when the repeal took effect, recalled, "I saw us in one day going from the Middle Ages to the modern world."

But beyond the mere fact of legality, this period of the late 1960s and early 1970s was genuinely exciting for these physicians because of the several innovations taking place. The introduction to a U.S. medical audience of the vacuum suction method, the invention and dissemination of the Karman cannula, and breakthroughs in modes of delivering local anesthesia all made abortion less risky for the physician to perform and less painful and costly for the patient. A new organizational form for the delivery of abortions – the freestanding clinic – was closely tied to these technical innovations.

These various innovations – and especially the development of the freestanding clinic – made for a heady atmosphere, in the immediate pre-*Roe* years, for those committed to abortion practice. For this group, for the first time, began to see the possibility of safe, accessible abortion for all their patients, *and*, for themselves, new terrain to develop as providers of legal abortion. Daniel Fieldstone recalls the tremendous energy he and his colleagues expended in that period. "We were just trying to provide them and make them safer and safer. And that was taking up all of our time and using up all of our energy. I was writing manuals. I wrote two manuals on abortion, and we were writing papers, chapters in books, and writing things all over the place on humane abortions."

Fieldstone recalls his early enthusiasm about the freestanding abortion clinic first in terms of decent patient care. "We saw freestanding clinics as a fantastic model for delivering medical services, because the well-run freestanding places were capable of not only providing less expensive services but also much more compassionate services than the hospitals. The hospitals were and still are inefficient and somewhat unpleasant, because you didn't recruit people who were essentially pro-woman, and pro-choice." But Fieldstone also saw the freestanding clinic as having the broader potential to pioneer in the emergent field of outpatient surgery: "The original idea was that abortion could be provided in freestanding centers that would also provide contraceptive services. As that settled down, we began to get into sterilization services. . . . [It became clear] that we can do some surgical services outside the hospital, freed of the weight of the bureaucracy and the cost of all those things, running the laundry, all those administrative services. You could be costeffective. . . . I think [freestanding abortion clinics] were the impetus for ambulatory surgery . . . hernias, hemorrhoids, whatever. A lot has changed since 1971, and the abortion movement, I think, helped streamline surgical services."

The freestanding clinics, however, proved ultimately to be a mixed blessing to the abortion movement. While such organizations undoubtedly provided (and continue to do so today) an effective, lowcost, and humanely delivered service, their very success – ironically – helped further the isolation of abortion services (and many abortion providers) from mainstream medicine – a dilemma to which I will return.

CHAPTER SIX

"Getting Your Hands Dirty":
The Practice of Legal Abortion

*We were doing abortions that day when the news came over the radio.
It was just an overwhelming feeling, I got tears in my eyes. . . . At last it
was all over, finally, . . . never again the fear, the threats, the violence,
[the threat of] going to prison, the constant harassment, fear of the
woman not being able to get service. It was a new day.* – DAVID BENNETT

*Then there was January 22 [1973]. January 22 I was at home, in bed,
with a cold. It was about ten in the morning. I was listening to the
radio and I heard the Supreme Court's decision. I could not believe
it! It was mind-boggling! I was thrilled. I was so excited I could
hardly stay in bed with my illness. That [decision] meant several
things to me, some on a very personal level. . . . It also provided an
opportunity for me; we no longer had to be restricted by the cost
constraints and the administrative constraints of the hospital. . . .
Now I had the opportunity to set up something [freestanding clinic]
which would be valuable for the community, a public service.*
– MARTY KAUFMAN

When Roe v. Wade *came along, I was so relieved because now
I could thumb my nose at anyone who gave me a hard time.
I remember the president of the hospital used to say, "I wish we
could get rid of those abortions, I hate those abortions."*
– MORRIS FISCHER

*It was like a ton of bricks coming off my shoulders. . . . When (*Roe*)
came out, I was literally walking with my feet off the ground. . . .
Such a triumph had been accomplished by people I didn't
even know.* – CALEB BARRINGTON

These comments express the elation felt by virtually everyone interviewed for this book about the historic ruling of the U.S. Supreme Court on January 22, 1973, which legalized abortion. At the time of

Roe, Bennett and Kaufman were practicing in states which had already liberalized their abortion laws. Nonetheless, for both men, this ruling was very significant. For Bennett, in particular, *Roe* served to validate his past record of extensive provision of illegal abortions. For both, moreover, the new ruling promised better quality of care. Women who had previously traveled from their own states to seek abortions in more liberal states would now presumably find abortions closer to home, with back-up care more readily available, if needed, after the abortion. Also, as Kaufman's comments suggest, the rulings of this historic day would further facilitate what was already in place in some locations – the freestanding abortion clinic as a new model of medical service delivery.[1]

Fischer's comments convey the enormous relief felt by the many abortion providers in the pre-*Roe* period who had been practicing in the "gray area" of hospital committee-approved abortions, never sure if antiabortion colleagues or an ambitious district attorney would decide to investigate "unjustified" abortions.

In the period immediately before *Roe*, Barrington had just returned to his New England birthplace and had made the decision to start an abortion practice, even if that meant, ultimately, that he would be arrested. His euphoria was shared by the many abortion-sympathetic physicians of that period who, having witnessed the results of illegal abortion, now could reasonably assume that they would no longer have to choose between the practice of good medicine and their own personal freedom.

As I shall document, the enormous optimism felt by this group at the time of *Roe* has sharply diminished over the years. Certainly, some of the benefits promised by this ruling have been realized, the most fundamental of these being that death and complication rates from abortion fell dramatically after legalization, and legal abortion today continues to be one of the safest of all surgical procedures.[2]

But two factors in particular – the marginalization of abortion practice from mainstream medicine, and the eventual rise of a militant antiabortion movement – have come to sour considerably the victory felt by this group over the *Roe* decision. The euphoria with which David Bennett recalled greeting the news of *Roe* in 1973 contrasts poignantly with the bitterness he expressed in the late 1980s about the situation of abortion providers. Acknowledging his naïveté at the time of *Roe*, Bennett said ruefully, "It was not a 'new day' as it turned out. . . . In fact it became more difficult, not easier. Since it's been legal, I've had much more personal harassment." The stigmatization of abortion practice – both within the medical profession and in society at large – from the time of *Roe* to the present is the story of this chapter.

THE COSTS OF ABORTION WORK

The difficulties abortion providers would eventually face in the era of legalization were not immediately apparent to many of those interviewed. Rather, these physicians quickly saw the benefits of the new ruling with respect to women's health. Even this group – far more attuned than other physicians to abortion issues – were stunned to learn how much more illegal abortion there had been in the pre-*Roe* period than they had previously thought. As Ron Ehrlich commented, "I don't think we realized what was going on, the full impact of what was going on out there . . . because [now] in the emergency room, you could spend ten nights in a row in the E.R. and not see a pregnant woman miscarrying, and then, we saw three and four a night . . . so obviously, many of them were started." Similarly, Ken Gordon expressed his astonishment upon realizing how little experience the residents currently under his supervision had with miscarriages in the emergency room. "*Now* I know that many of those we thought were 'genuine' miscarriages really were not."

To be sure, some of those interviewed encountered institutional resistance immediately upon the passage of *Roe* and had to continue their advocacy activity. Eugene Fox, like several others, was driven to consider legal action to pressure his own hospital to conform to the new law. "In 1973, when the Supreme Court decision came down, I was no longer acting as chair of our department. We had a new younger chairman and I bulldozed him by threatening a lawsuit because he wouldn't have an abortion facility. He succumbed on that." When asked if he requested support from colleagues over this threatened lawsuit, Fox replied, "I had verbal support from several people, but they were like, 'I'll hold your coat, you get in there and fight.'"

In the mid-1970s, Morris Fischer returned from two years of practicing medicine abroad and assumed a professorship of obstetrics and gynecology in a medical school on the East Coast. "When I started work here, I started scheduling abortions. They told me, 'You are not allowed to do abortions in this institution.' I said, 'What are you talking about? This is 1975! *Roe v. Wade* was 1973!' . . . 'Well, we have a rule on our books.' 'Well, you can have a rule on your books that I am not going to stay here. You want my services, you want my talents, you say I am a big gun or something, then you have to have me as I am.' That very meeting when I spoke they put a motion up and it was ruled that I could do them up to and including twelve weeks but nothing beyond that. . . . They wanted to make it very clear that I wouldn't make the hospital into an abortion mill."

In some hospitals, even when the letter of the new law was obeyed, a combination of residual opposition to abortion and downright confusion as to how to implement this new service made the abortion highly unpleasant for the patient and the attending physician. Miriam Harkin recalled with distaste her first experience of attempting a hospital-based abortion in the immediate aftermath of *Roe*. "I can remember the first patient I took there to do a legal abortion, a day or two after *Roe v. Wade*. The good part was that she didn't have to go through this laborious approval committee. But she was sitting in the ward, waiting to have her abortion; the nurses would come to the door, peer at her, and make gestures of disapproval. . . . So the woman was waiting, I was waiting, the whole afternoon. Finally, the hospital administrator comes up and says we can't do this, the details of the law haven't been worked out. We had to go to another hospital, and I didn't get to do her until around five or six o'clock because we had been mucking around all day. What a hassle."

It was precisely the "hassles" that Harkin and others experienced in their hospitals that made the freestanding clinic so attractive. The excitement felt by many of those interviewed about the abortion clinic was that here, finally, abortion patients would be treated with some decency. As Harkin put it, "I felt it was so important to have special freestanding clinics, where there are caring people, not general medical people, not self-righteous people. Our Victorian morality has been antiabortion for so long, that even people – like the nurses –

who are otherwise kind and caring can be so cruel in the abortion situation."

As discussed in the previous chapter, the initial enthusiasm many abortion providing physicians felt about the freestanding clinic was also because of its innovative character as a health delivery model. As such, participating in the creation and refinement of this model offered to some the possibility of both a professional challenge and a means of upgrading the image of abortion. Barry Messinger reminisced about his decision to continue to be intensely involved in abortion work after *Roe*, particularly his leadership in establishing a freestanding clinic in his community: "I guess I'm a maverick. . . . I like to do things that are different. It was a new territory. . . . I had already been involved in dealing with women's reproduction in a number of different ways and here was a new way to help them. And it was a way to kind of show my more conservative colleagues that something new could be added to medicine, and it was going to work. And it was reputable and good."

Ethan Stevenson was just completing his residency in obstetrics/gynecology in New England when *Roe v. Wade* was decided. He then worked for several years at one of the several Preterm clinics that were being established in that period. The original Preterm freestanding abortion clinic had been established in 1971 in Washington, D.C. by Harry Levin, formerly of the Population Council. The Washington facility quickly became the largest single center for abortions outside New York state and also became very influential in setting standards for abortion care across the country. Many physicians, both in the United States and abroad, came to the Washington facility to learn the techniques of performing abortions.[5] The Preterm model, moreover, emphasized integrating abortion counseling, contraceptive services, sexual counseling, and, eventually, sterilization services with abortion services. A series of eight Preterm manuals on the various aspects of establishing a freestanding abortion clinic became widely distributed throughout the country in the period immediately after *Roe*.

Stevenson's experiences at a Preterm clinic are illustrative of both the advantages and, ultimately, the limitations, of full-time work in such a setting for the abortion-providing physician. On the positive side, Stevenson became involved in influential circles of abortion innovators, encountering people who remain valued mentors and colleagues to this day. Although he had some experience with abortion as a resident, he nonetheless insisted on visiting the flagship Preterm clinic in Washington, D.C. to receive further training in abortion technique. The Preterm at which he worked similarly had an air of excitement and innovation. "The Preterm I was at was a very exciting place in those times. There was a community board, a wonderful and interesting group of people . . . folks on the cutting edge. Harry Levin [Preterm's founder] had perfected his lay counselor model in Washington and was introducing that everywhere else."

In the several years he spent full time at Preterm – with half his days spent doing abortions and the other half working on the contraceptive service – Stevenson honed his skills. As was common everywhere in the early days of legal abortion, some physicians simply were technically more proficient than others – both causing less pain to the patient and having a lower injury rate. At Preterm, Stevenson worked with one other full-time abortion provider, Dr. Belize [not his real name] and, as Stevenson put it, "I kept having to bail him out of trouble. . . . He'd have technical difficulties. Also he also had real trouble talking to the patients or the counselors. The thing about counselors is that they quite quickly figure out who is good and who isn't, and they are patient advocates. They were *supposed* to be patient advocates. So they would come around and say, 'Listen, this patient is going to be tough to do, will you do her? I don't want Dr. Belize to do her.' "

But although Stevenson had the satisfaction of being known as the superior abortion provider, and generally had the respect of the counselors, he gradually came to find his work in some respects ungratifying. In his words, "I began to feel like the fool at the end of the curette." Stevenson is here referring to the highly specialized role – that of "technician" as many refer to it – that doctors came to play in these early clinics – and in most clinics still do today. This specialization carries with it a certain bureaucratic logic, but often comes at the price of physician alienation, if not burnout. As Stevenson explained the early management rationale for the sharp demarcation of the physician's role from those of others in the clinic: "They [doctors] are expensive tools and should be used for what only they could do, and everything else should be done by people that cost less."

A small but significant body of research that was done in the first years of legal abortion resonates with Stevenson's experiences. A number of researchers found that attitudes toward abortion work were more positive among groups such as social workers and lay counselors who had extended verbal contact with the patient than among physicians and nurses. The argument is that those who had more experience with the "whole" woman were more likely to focus on her and see the procedure in light of her particular situation – in contrast to doctors and nurses who dealt with the more physically unpleasant aspects of abortion, without any mitigating sense of the individual patient.[4]

In the period he worked at Preterm, Stevenson took several steps to, as he put it, "work himself out of the job of being the fool at the end of the curette" and to make his abortion activity more gratifying. First came the realization that he could manage to have more of a relationship with the abortion recipient. "It worked out that there was a bit of room to amplify my own interaction with the patients, and I remember thinking at the time that each abortion is like a performance. It's like being on stage for this woman right now. Quickly form a little bit of a relationship and do my best to make this not an unpleasant thing for her. Establish warmth and friendliness and support and do the procedure as best as I could and be as nice as I could to her in this very limited period of time."

His second strategy was to redouble his efforts to glean whatever knowledge he could from the clinic experience. "What I wanted to do was to develop what there was of the potential spirit of science. Learn from what was going on. I would have loved to have more guidance doing that. And eventually I began to get it from Dave Fields [not his real name] who had been hired to be medical director of the Preterm Institute, in Washington. And he did come to [our clinic] some. That was really wonderful. Here was somebody I could admire and respect who was doing this work and a serious person, but a nice person. It was very important to me."

But Stevenson's attempts to incorporate more "scientific" aspects into his work routine were not wholly successful. Though a number of the first generation of innovators of the freestanding clinic wrote influential papers on the delivery of abortion services to a large volume of patients, Stevenson's efforts were discouraged by his clinic director. "One of my great disappointments – I put together a paper on my first ten thousand abortions and got it ready to send off and presented it to him, and he said, 'What do you want to do that for? Why do you want to write a paper?'" Stevenson speculated that he was discouraged from medical research because his supervisor felt it would detract too much from his clinic work.

Similarly, the possibility to do international work was only partially realized for Stevenson at Preterm. Stevenson had had a deep interest in international population issues since his adolescence and had hoped to become engaged in work in the developing world. "Now I had expected that Preterm was going to develop into an international institution, and my own vision of what would happen is that I would be at Preterm half time and then I would go over to the Preterm Institute and get to work on helping to develop the international stuff. But I misunderstood the economics. There just wasn't the money to do it. They [preterm management] really needed me doing what I was doing." Stevenson did manage one international trip during this period, which was sponsored by another organization, the Pathfinder Fund. He went to the Caribbean with an experienced Preterm counselor and introduced various regional health officials there to the method of suction curettage, done under local anesthesia, as well as to the concept of counseling the abortion recipient.

Significantly, Stevenson came to realize that full-time work at a freestanding clinic, immediately after his residency, might block his future career development. "I negotiated with Preterm to let me work one day a week at the hospital. . . . By then they had created the hospital abortion service. I worked on that service with residents and I also stayed that night, as the junior attending for the residents on the delivery floor, so that kept me involved with regular obstetrics. And allowed me to get my boards. You have to practice for two years after you take your written boards and present your case list, and I would never have been able to get boards if I had just been doing outpatient abortions. I'm not sure I fully understood that when I went to work for Preterm, but I quite quickly realized that I couldn't at that point in my career just do that, or I would go nowhere."

To be sure, each of the physicians interviewed for this study has a unique configuration of personal characteristics and career contingencies that helps explain his or her current assessment of abortion work, but in Stevenson's reflections on his early experience in a freestanding clinic, we can find suggestions of some general dilemmas inherent in this work. A major problem of abortion work, as it has developed since 1973, is that for most practitioners there is little professional challenge in it once the basic technique of suction curettage has been mastered. It is true, as I have documented, that for some of the pioneers active in the period immediately before and after *Roe* it was an exciting time of innovation in both techniques and service delivery models.[5] But most providers, even some of the "pioneers" I have cited, came to acknowledge the routinization of most abortion work. This routinization has contributed to abortion provision's relative lack of status in the larger medical community – and especially within the world of obstetrics and gynecology. Barry Messinger, himself one of the most influential of abortion innovators, spoke quite candidly about the limitations of abortion specialization as a career for those in academic medicine. Commenting on the period surrounding *Roe,* he said, "I knew that not very many of my academic colleagues were interested or willing to put time into doing abortions. . . . I also became aware of the fact that the technique was rapidly becoming simple and one would not be able to write a lot of papers about its complexities and its advances and permutations – things like that. So from that point of view, it's not a very intellectually challenging deal . . . and I think one would have had to be in early, like I was, to make certain contributions. And also it would help if one were kind of sociologically dedicated to the proposition that women should have this as part of their medical care. And I think that limited the kind of academic people who would be interested in it."

Judith Harmon, in speaking of the reluctance of mainstream physicians to become involved with the freestanding clinic movement –

both immediately after *Roe* and in the present – gave an even more explicitly feminist twist to her analysis. "Definitely then, and even maybe more so today, the academic people saw you couldn't afford to get your hands dirty with this stuff unless you were an extremely powerful person and just happened to be enough of a humanist.... You know, a lower-level person couldn't possibly risk contaminating their career.... It is not intellectual, that's for sure.... I don't think it's all that different from any of the other 'women's issues,' even in ob/gyn it's not actually okay to *care* about women in that kind of way.... You can only care intellectually about pituitary tumors in women.... It's kind of like being interested in daycare or something! I think the same is true about contraception ... things like barrier method, condoms or diaphragms, who would care about that? It's too ordinary."

Daniel Fieldstone, himself a professor in a medical school, assessed the status of abortion specialists in very blunt terms: "There is virtually no chair [in departments of obstetrics and gynecology] whose career was made around contraception, sterilization, and abortion.... These are really regarded as trivial issues in ob/gyn. Molecular genetics, endocrinology, steroid chemistry, cell biology on the academic scale are considered to be more important than this kind of thing."

If abortion-sympathetic physicians seeking to establish a career in academic medicine found that abortion specialization was considered low status, those more fully committed to private practice found that even after *Roe* their work as abortion providers still carried much emotional baggage. Some of their colleagues made quite clear how distasteful the image of the "abortionist" was. As Eugene Fox said, "Even my own colleagues there at University Hospital, I would be over there delivering a baby, and they would say, 'What are you doing here? I didn't think you delivered babies, I thought you just did abortions'.... Some of my colleagues don't speak to me because I do abortions." Similarly, Bob Phillips felt his other contributions to medicine over a long career became slighted by colleagues fixated on the abortion issue. "Well, you know, every now and then you get labeled an 'abortionist,' which is a term I don't really enjoy.... At a medical meeting, something like that, as soon as you become identified with the [pro-choice] movement, you become an 'abortionist.' Now that to me is an unpleasant term because I'm no more an abortionist than I am an obstetrician or a hysterectomist or any other procedure that I do. 'Abortionist' carries a still unpleasant connotation. It carries the connotation of a sleaze."

Some physicians who began doing abortions after legalization came into conflict with partners who were uneasy about such activity. Charles Swensen, a particularly visible spokesman for abortion in his state, spoke of such a conflict with his partners in a large group practice. "The senior partners were in principle supportive of abortion but they did not like the notoriety that I as an individual was receiving in the press, and as a result they docked my income by about 15 percent. . . . We had a meeting and they said, 'Okay, we've calculated this, and this is where we are setting your percentage of remuneration that will come for the next four years.' I said, 'What can I do to improve that for the next go-around?" and they said, 'Well, you should get out of the abortion business.' "

But if practitioners who combined abortion work with other activities suffered a certain chilly reception from colleagues, the ostracism felt by those who chose full-time abortion work is even more evident. David Bennett spoke with bitterness about the difficult relations he had with various sectors of the medical community in the period immediately after *Roe.* In attempting to establish a nonprofit abortion clinic and get local physicians who would both serve on the board and perform abortions, Bennett found that his history as a provider of illegal abortion tainted his image among his would-be colleagues. "There were some who said they'd be willing to provide abortion service with such a set-up but they didn't want to have anything to do with me. . . . It was because I was an 'abortionist.' . . . An abortionist is a despicable person. They assumed you did it for the money, you didn't have the qualifications to be a real doctor . . . you were either a drug addict, an alcoholic, a ne'er do well, you couldn't maintain a practice or you were owned by the Mafia. . . . You weren't a good person and probably weren't a good doctor either. At the very least, you were an embarrassment to the medical community."

Similarly, when Bennett moved to a new community and attempted to join the local county medical society (a necessary step to gaining hospital privileges in that area), his application generated considerable controversy. Though some of his colleagues supported him very strongly, others just as strongly opposed his membership. Again, his history of providing illegal abortion was an issue, particularly the fact that he acknowledged having broken the law – though as Bennett and his supporters argued, as an act of civil disobedience he had broken a law that subsequently was declared unconstitutional. "Well, finally this committee [credential committee] recommended my membership, but there was so much opposition, I had to go the meeting. There are doctors who are standing up and saying such things as, 'He's a murderer and not fit to sit among us.' I had to sit and listen to all of this tirade." Bennett feels that had he not been able to produce a letter of recommendation from the head of the department of obstetrics and gynecology at a respected medical school (who had referred patients to him), his application would not have been approved.

Many of those interviewed for this study were also able to point to various penalties imposed by colleagues that appeared to be a direct consequence of their involvement in abortion. Ed Lever and Daniel Fieldstone, both in academic medicine, have ample reason to suspect that certain career promotions were sabotaged because of the abortion issue. Lever spoke of the particular wrath his pro-choice stand evoked in his former mentor, Dr. Morgan. "Dr. Morgan became so angry with me because of my views on the abortion issue and the civil rights issue. . . . At one of the legislative sessions where he was present, he stood up in front of the legislative hearing board and said, 'I will see to it that your reputation is ruined in this community.'" Lever's reaction to this public denunciation was a fear that proved well founded. "I had moved up from clinical instructor to a clinical associate, and then one day the man in the department who was responsible for the advancement of the clinical faculty said to me, 'I think you've done enough stuff, I think we should make you a full professor, would you be interested?' I said, 'I would be honored.' It never happened and I found out later that it didn't happen because Dr. Morgan (who was retired) had enough power to hold my appointment back. I was told there were ways I could change that. I said, 'I'm not interested.' I didn't want to have to do something which was against my better judgment and principles, and what they really wanted me to do was to go easy on the abortion issue, stop being in the limelight. I said, 'I don't choose to be in the limelight but I'm medical director of the clinic and when media interviews are necessary, it's my job to do them.' "

Similarly, Daniel Fieldstone perceives his high visibility as an abortion advocate as an impediment in the professional culture of academic medicine. "I've never been asked to be a chair. . . . I'm viewed as being so heavily involved in the abortion issue – I am probably too controversial for most medical schools. As a matter of fact, though I have no proof of it, I suspect it's a good part of why I didn't get tenure at this school."

Charles Swensen can directly link his repudiation by an exclusive professional association to his abortion work.

I was invited to apply to join the so-called prestigious Pacific Coast Ob/ Gyn Society about ten years ago. . . . This is invitation only, and the local caucus [from Swensen's own community] that are members of the society make a recommendation to the general membership. There were a significant number of those [caucus] members who are right-to-lifers, who blackballed my name. Usually they invite you to go to a meeting, you go to a meeting, they look at you, if they like you they invite you back to give a paper, and if they like the paper, you're a member. Well, I wasn't invited back. I got a phone call one day from a friend of mine who had proposed me. . . . He told me he had become incensed about the situation and had gone to find out about it, what was going on, he was going to do all he could to turn that around, and about two years later I got a kind of very apologetic letter that sort of indicated that an oversight had occurred, and they apologized for not inviting me back, would I consider coming back. By that time, I was involved in so many damn things that it was five more years before I could find time in my schedule to go, and of course now I'm a member in good standing.

Ron Ehrlich, a highly respected and energetic physician – involved in a broad spectrum of obstetrical issues – had every reason to believe he was going to be made chief of the department of obstetrics and gynecology in his renowned suburban hospital. However, his work in a freestanding abortion clinic apparently derailed his appointment.

> The chairman of our department became ill and had to very quickly retire. And there were two people who were made temporary chairmen, myself and the present chairman, who is a good friend of mine. And we both went to interviews . . . they had a search committee. Only two candidates. And there wasn't a human being in the hospital that didn't automatically believe that I would be chief – not a person. Not an aide, not a maid, not a person that didn't say, "You'll be chief," "when you're chief" . . . and I was not made chief. And in the interview, in a very nonaccusatory way . . . they said, "Well, you're still involved with that clinic?" And then I went to someone who was a very good friend of mine, who was chairman of another department, and I said, "I want you to tell me why I wasn't made chief; I want to know," and she as much as said to me, "mostly because of the abortion issue."
>
> It's not something I really wanted . . . you think you don't want it, but when it's right there for you to have, you say, "Boy, I'd like to be chief." The person that was made chief is not as capable as I am, and he lacks a lot of the qualities that one needs in a chief. So he asked me if I would be chief of obstetrics, under him, and I accepted that. And so I have sort of a role. And there are times when people come to me and don't go to him, which he doesn't resent at all. We have a nice relationship. He's a wonderful guy.

As a final example of being held back or punished for being involved in abortion, Caleb Barrington, who had tried to arrange approved abortions for nurses and army dependents while he served in the military, reported: "I was seen as an agitator. I was the only guy that wasn't decorated out of my group of ob/gyns. It was because of abortion."

In reflecting upon the professional costs of abortion involvement, several caveats are in order. First, it is obviously impossible to draw definitive conclusions when the only evidence available is the respondents' self-reports. It is of course plausible that some of these professional slights were, in fact, due to other factors. Furthermore, some of the doctors interviewed for this book are counterexamples, physicians who were given affirmation and positions of responsibility by their peers despite their abortion practice. For example, when I questioned Ken Gordon, who for many years had been a highly vocal spokesman for abortion rights in his large East Coast city, about any professional costs associated with abortion, he replied, "The best answer I can give you is that a couple of years ago I was elected president of the Valley Obstetrical and Gynecological Society. I would say that there were about twenty to thirty or so right-to-life ob/gyns in this area who won't talk to me, and my feeling about that is, thank God! The obstetrical/gynecological society in this area has about four hundred members and I never felt unwelcome there." Similarly, Harris Bishop, one of the handful of abortion providers in his highly conservative state, was chosen by his peers to be chief of obstetrics at his hospital. Paul Temple, who has been a target of extensive antiabortion activity in his Midwest city, was elected by his colleagues – also in a quite conservative community – to serve on the executive committee of his hospital and was also honored by his peers for his achievements as a family physician. George Jacobs has held one of the highest elective offices within the major professional association for most of those interviewed, the American College of Obstetricians and Gynecologists. And notwithstanding Fieldstone's comments about those highly identified with abortion being blackballed in academic medicine, a number of major medical institutions in the United States – among them, Harvard, Columbia, and the University of California at San Francisco – have had department heads and deans who were eminent researchers and teachers in the area of abortion.

Finally, to reiterate, even those who report the most clearcut examples of having been "punished" for abortion activity are nonetheless, by any conventional measure, successful physicians. All those interviewed in this study suggested that they had busy professional lives, and all appeared to be earning a comfortable living.

Notwithstanding abortion providers' periodic confrontations with antiabortion doctors, if polls are to be believed, the majority of their physician colleagues support legal abortion. This majority is, obviously, dependent on them in making abortion referrals. (In fact, among those referring to abortion providers are physicians who label themselves "antiabortion."[6]) But, as many of those interviewed suggested, "referrals" are not always indicative of true collegiality. In many ways – some subtle and some not so subtle – those who provide abortions are often made to feel that they are outsiders in the medical community. This odd combination of dependency and superiority on the part of colleagues who do not do abortions is wryly amusing to some providers and highly exasperating to others. Paul Temple performs abortions later in pregnancy than many other providers, and thus receives numerous patients from out of town. This activity has generated considerable flak over the years from some local physicians, but Temple maintains his equanimity and speaks of his "evolving" relationship with his colleagues in these terms: "See, some of the physicians that were giving me all the heat were my contemporaries, and they are finding life is not all black and white like they thought it was. Some of them are maturing in their thinking.... There are lots of people who love us, but don't want to do [abortions] themselves.... They're certainly happy that I'm well trained, but they don't want to get their hands dirty – and that's okay."

Victor Black, who operates his own freestanding clinic, spoke similarly of his perception of his status among his medical peers. "I'm sure there are some gynecologists in the area who would say, 'That guy doesn't do anything but abortions.' On the other hand, I have many gynecologists who refer to me – they are very fine gynecologists – but they don't want to do abortions themselves, largely because of their staff. Some nursing staffs don't want to do abortions if they are only going to do one or two a month. They just don't want to do it. So, these doctors refer to me. I have patients who come in and say, 'Dr. So and So said if I am going to have this done, I should only go to you.'... My reputation in this community, for what I do, is top notch." Irving Goodman carried this "dependency" notion a step further when, in response to a question of whether he felt his colleagues in his hospital "respected" him, he answered laughingly, "They'd better! Since at least half this hospital has been through my office. If I called a general strike of everybody in my area that has been through this office, we would close the economy down! And this goes from very high up, to all the way down."

But for some, particularly those whose medical practice is solely or largely devoted to abortions, referrals from other physicians do not signify the collegial affirmation that is so important in a professional career. This is the case with David Bennett, whose difficulties in joining his local medical society shortly after *Roe* were discussed earlier. Though with the passage of time, Bennett has secured a place within the medical establishment in his southwestern community – that is, he has privileges at several local hospitals and operates two successful freestanding clinics which offer abortion and gynecological services – he is still acutely aware of the abortion provider's marginal status. Speaking of the lack of regard from colleagues, he said, "If you walk down the halls of that hospital, you're not going to hear anyone say, 'There goes David Bennett, he's the famous abortionist.' ... They're not going to put up any plaques for the abortionist in the medical society or the hospital."

The stigmatization of abortion services – and the subtle reprisals against the abortion provider that often accompany it – is thus pervasive in contemporary medical practice. Sometimes the stigma is felt as a status wound by the individual practitioner, as in the above example of David Bennett, or when, as some providers report, even friendly colleagues "jokingly" refer to them as "baby killers." Sometimes, more consequentially, this stigma is apparent in the ongoing struggles providers have to wage over such matters as their hospitals' willingness to establish and maintain abortion services and to serve as back-up facilities for freestanding clinics – matters that many thought would have been long settled some twenty years after the *Roe* decision. Most seriously, though, given the bitter opposition of some of their medical colleagues, abortion providers have come to fear both medical reprisals against their patients and legal reprisals against themselves. For example, at a 1992 meeting on the management of complications of clinic-based abortions, when the question arose of sending a patient with a perforation to the hospital, one speaker voiced his concern about the possibility of an antiabortion doctor performing a "punitive hysterectomy." Providers of clinic

abortions speak of other seemingly unnecessary and expensive procedures to which their patients are subjected if complications arise
after the women have returned to their hometowns; for example, in
the case of retained tissue, which typically would only require resuc-
tioning, some women have been hospitalized and made to undergo
what abortion providers feel are unwarranted D.& C.'s – a medical
"overreaction" which abortion physicians attribute to antiabortion
zeal.[7] Furthermore, the already embroiled legal climate in which
many of these physicians operate – ob/gyns have among the highest
rates of malpractice suits[8] – is further complicated by the willingness of antiabortion physicians to aggressively participate in legal actions against abortion providers.

The dilemma facing contemporary abortion providers, therefore,
might be summed up as follows: these providers are strongly opposed by a highly energized minority within medicine; rather pas-
sively tolerated by the majority; and actively supported only by a relative few. It is a predicament in which the collegiality that is such a
crucial aspect of medical practice – and which has implications ranging from the most personal, such as self-validation, to the pragmatic,
such as the management of medical emergencies – is often elusive for
abortion providers. This lack of proactive support from medical colleagues in turn reflects how much has *not* occurred within the institutional structures of U.S. medicine with respect to abortion provision. Put most simply, U.S. medicine has not normalized the practice
of abortion since the *Roe* decision in 1973.

To be sure, as I have already suggested, the marginality of abortion providers is in part the result of the very success of pro-choice
physicians and others in developing the freestanding abortion clinic.
This innovation has enabled women to obtain abortions at a lower
cost, with less discomfort, and, arguably, with more humane treatment than would be received in a hospital. But originally, as concep-
tualized by Jane Hodgson and other abortion innovators of the early
1970s, the freestanding clinic was to have a very close working relationship with mainstream medicine. Besides readily accepting those
occasional patients that needed hospitalization, it was hoped that
hospitals would send their ob/gyn residents to the clinics to receive

training in abortion procedures, that the leading ob/gyns of the community would themselves provide some hours of service there, that the clinics would serve as a research base for academic medicine, and so on. Furthermore, the clinic founders never intended the clinics to be virtually the *only* settings for abortion services in many communities (leading to situations in which, because of opposition from the local medical establishment, doctors servicing the clinic are flown in from out of town, and the hospital agreeing to provide back-up service for the clinic is miles away). Rather, what the first generation of legal abortion providers envisioned was a complex of services: in addition to clinics, it was assumed that most trained ob/gyns would perform some abortions in their offices, and that hospitals would rapidly develop services for later and more difficult abortions – as well as outpatient clinics for earlier abortions in communities that had no freestanding facility. Yet very little of this original vision has been realized. Perhaps the greatest indication of the failure of the medical establishment to respond to the abortion needs of women is the lack of abortion facilities in hospitals in areas which have no clinics. At present, only 7 percent of all abortions in the United States take place in a hospital.[9]

While the dramatic, violent assaults on clinic facilities and abortion providers by antiabortionists have dominated headlines since the late 1980s and are commonly viewed as the chief reason for physicians' withdrawal from abortion, in fact much of the medical establishment had already distanced itself from abortion services in the years before antiabortion violence began to escalate – mainly by supporting legal abortion in principle, while refusing to take part in the practice of abortion. The latter-day rise of antiabortion activism, to which I now turn, has only exacerbated an already precarious situation.

ANTIABORTION HARASSMENT AND ABORTION PRACTICE

As an antiabortion movement mobilized and expanded in the United States in the years after *Roe*, abortion-providing physicians increasingly began to be harassed at their workplaces and homes. Since the

late 1980s, with the emergence of Operation Rescue and similar
groups, the violence and terrorism against abortion providers has increased dramatically, leading some researchers to speak of an "epidemic" of antiabortion violence in this country.[10] Nearly all of those
interviewed for this study have been subject to hostile actions by antiabortionists, though the severity of these actions – and thus, the impact upon the professional and personal lives of the respondents –
varies considerably. Also, the reader should bear in mind that most
of the interviews for this study were completed just before the sharp
escalation in violence against abortion providers in the United States.
Among those who are quoted in the pages that follow, one physician
was shot (though only slightly wounded) outside his office, subsequent to our interview, and another had to cope with hundreds of Operation Rescue activists surrounding his house as part of a national
campaign to harass providers in their homes. Yet another respon-
dent, since being interviewed, has become embroiled in a struggle
with antiabortion activists in his conservative state who are trying to
close down his office on a legal technicality. Several have had their
offices firebombed, forcing them to relocate.

The most common form of antiabortion activity is to picket a
clinic or doctor's office. In most cases, though it can be extremely
annoying to both provider and patient, over time this picketing gets
routinized – that is, often the same small group of picketers will turn
out at predictable times and become known factors to the doctors and
their staff.[11] As Horace Freeman, the medical director of a large freestanding clinic on the East Coast, put it, "We have a cop here every
day. We have marches every day, every single day. Only like three or
four people, and we started to get used to them, and they got used to
us. 'Good morning, doctor, have you changed your mind? Remember,
doctor, you are killing babies.' ... I get in my car and drive off. I find
little stickers they leave on my bumper."

Oswald Watson, a retired physician who moved to the West Coast
and was retrained as an abortion provider, takes in stride his daily
confrontation with picketers and confesses to sometimes enjoying
responding to their taunts. "I go through the picket lines – according
to them, here's an old gray-haired bastard, they couldn't get too

worked up. I remember one time one of the right-to-lifers in the picket line said, 'You just can't make enough money, can you?' I said, 'No, you hit it right on the head.'"

Bill Swinton, practicing in a small town in the Pacific Northwest, went the farthest of all those interviewed to find "common ground" with his regular band of picketers.[12] "The first pickets were quite a surprise to us. It was a fundamentalist group and they did it haphazardly, and then they started every Friday at noon. Someone came and told us one of the local doctors' wives had joined them. The way we dealt with it was very benignly. I was willing to talk to them. One time they were picketing us, and it was getting to be Christmastime, and we decided we'll get a bunch of cider and some cookies, and we didn't schedule anybody for that Friday noon. We kept a wide open space. Well, we got all the cider and things ready and they didn't come that day!"

But if most picketers are known factors and ultimately not physically dangerous, there is a chronic, well-founded concern among providers that, without notice, picketing will escalate to violence. Horace Freeman, quoted above on the predictable nature of his "regulars," went on to add: "But there are days when they get itchy.... I mean, one morning we had twelve come in and chain themselves to the beds. We took them to court, they were all convicted and fined, and were told if they ever did it again they would go to jail."

Zachary Harris's clinic was firebombed, causing extensive damage. Speaking of the suspect, Harris said, "Well, he's arrested and charged, and he'll be prosecuted, but I don't know what will happen. I think all that does is simply add to the public perception that the antiabortion people are crazy and will stop at nothing.... They're a bunch of lunatics and every time there's something like that, it evokes a little more sympathy from the community toward what we're doing. I think it's totally counterproductive." Harris, however, continually receives threatening phone calls and letters, is subjected to regular demonstrations at his clinic, and currently performs abortions behind a wall of extra-thick plate glass, sometimes wearing a bulletproof vest.

Disruptions inside the clinic itself are, of course, chaotic – potentially nightmarish – situations. Caleb Barrington, who claimed that for several years he had actually enjoyed bantering with the small group who regularly picketed the Planned Parenthood clinic where he worked as medical director, described a far more serious incident. The incident occurred, according to Barrington, after the local anti-abortion group had been trained by a more militant national group in the techniques of closing down abortion facilities.

> They found a young woman at the university who came to the clinic one day, said she was pregnant. The counselor talked to her there for awhile and tried to get her to have an exam. She said she had to get to school, and so the counselor asked for a urine specimen; she said she'd try, but she couldn't get a urine specimen. The counselor said, "Well, if you are pregnant, how do you feel about it?" She said she wasn't sure, she was going to go home and think some more. . . . So the counselor said, "Well okay, our next abortion clinic is on Tuesday, why don't you come in about eight o'clock on Tuesday morning?" So she came at 8:00 and about 8:15 a group of people charged into the clinic, cameras flashing, took pictures of everybody there, came in with press cameras and blocked the door to all the abortion offices, saying, "We are saving babies and we are not going to let these people go on murdering people. This is a citizens' arrest. . . . We're not trespassing because we are here stopping a crime." The clinic called the police, the police came in, they called me, and I arrived there. Finally, the police ordered them to leave and they wouldn't, so they started to handcuff them all. The trouble was that the press was there and I didn't want these people to look like martyrs . . . because a couple of the police were getting quite rough. I said, "I don't want any pictures of you guys being rough with people in our clinic, and I want all of these people to be treated humanely."
>
> So they all went to jail. A couple of them refused to pay bail and stayed in jail right through to the trial. . . . The prosecutor, who was just prosecuting for trespassing, was Catholic himself and allowed them to use the trial as a scathing indictment against Planned Parenthood and as a forum on when life begins and all that. And the judge comes in grumbling, and he had to keep chiding the so-called prosecutor for letting all this stuff go on. Normally, the prosecutor would object that it wasn't relevant, but the judge had to do it himself. In the trial this young

woman that had come to our clinic swore that we were going to do an abortion on her without a pregnancy test and without having done an exam when she wasn't even pregnant. One of the charges she had was that she wasn't properly counselled and that Planned Parenthood did abortions just on anybody who came in off the street whether they were pregnant or not. . . . I was really angry, but it was fun to watch the testimony because we were able to show that Planned Parenthood was not doing abortions that morning but had brought her in four hours early to make sure she had time to talk to the counselor, have her exam and urine test, and that she wasn't going to have an abortion at 8:15 as she thought, because there was no one there to do it then. I wasn't scheduled to arrive until 1:00 in the afternoon. We were lucky in a way that we weren't doing abortions that morning. All the other people in the clinic then were these young teenagers coming in for birth control, some without parental consent, and they all disappeared when these people arrived in the clinic with their cameras. I am sure it was scary for them.

Such clinic disruptions have additional effects, beyond the obvious stress they cause staff and patients who are present at the time of the incident. The publicity they generate affects both current and potential patients of the abortion provider. Barrington claimed that when he first began to provide abortions at his own office, immediately after the *Roe* decision, the presence of picketers was – ironically – helpful. "They would stage a picket at the office and would at the same time make it a media event. They would call the press, they would all arrive, and the next day I would get twice as many phone calls because people would know I was doing abortions – so, in fact, they made my name known."

Today, though, the presence of antiabortionists outside the clinic and office are at best an annoyance, and at worst, a factor that drives some patients away. Some patients leave a doctor's general practice because of their principled opposition to abortion. As Ron Ehrlich stated, "If for some reason I make the newspapers, because they picket or something, I will get perhaps half a dozen phone calls in the next two weeks from people who were, for some reason, oblivious to the fact [that he performed abortions]. And they will call and say, 'I've been your patient for many years and I think you're terrific, but I can't come back anymore? So we know that . . . there are some people who don't come [to physicians who also provide abortions] and some who leave. . . . The bottom line is, I couldn't be busier than I am." Other patients avoid such offices on more practical grounds. Harris Bishop stated it bluntly: "You lose a certain amount of patients that don't want to put up with the hassle of walking through a picket line."

Antiabortion protests not only have the potential to drive away some patients, but also make recruiting medical staff more complicated. Ron Ehrlich, who maintains an extremely active obstetrical/gynecological practice, has a policy of only bringing in partners who are also willing to work some shifts at the abortion clinic he directs. "Now this fellow that joined us, Gary, he joined me three years ago, and he knew we did abortions, because he had worked for me at the clinic years ago. And when he came into the practice, he knew he had to continue to do that. And he would park two blocks away. And he didn't want anybody to know he worked there, and he didn't want his name on a prescription blank, and he didn't want his name on the wall."

Antiabortionists' intrusion into the professional lives of abortion providers takes forms other than picketing. Eugene Fox had to contend with antiabortion activists telephoning his patients "to tell them that I kill babies and stuff like that." Ed Lever told of an incident in which he and other abortion providers in his community were targeted by the local Catholic newspaper. "They ran a series of articles detailing the lives of the abortionists in the community. They got the information because of abortions we did on AFDC women with public funds. That was public information so they could find out from the welfare department how many abortions were done on public patients . . . the numbers, the patient, and the physician and the amount of money paid to us for doing it. . . . A suit was begun by us. The American Civil Liberties Union took the case . . . but according to state rule, that was public information."

Stan Ogden was involved in a somewhat similar case. He and a colleague were the major abortion providers at a publicly funded HMO (health maintenance organization) for which they worked. An antiabortion group demanded to know the names of those who had received abortions, and Ogden's organization was on the verge of complying. "I fought our organization because they were getting ready to give them the names and I said, 'You give them and I will personally sue the hell out of you.' We kept them at bay a while longer."

A number of those interviewed for this book are picketed and otherwise harassed at home. Ed Lever, a Jew who fled Nazi Germany, had a swastika painted on his house by antiabortionists, in addition to being regularly picketed. Some of those picketed at their homes, such as Miriam Harkin, found unexpected support from their neighbors, even those not known to be pro-choice. Harkin, a divorcee, lives in a suburb of "old die-hard conservatives" and is "usually not invited to the neighborhood parties." On the several occasions, however, that antiabortionists invaded her neighborhood, replete with bullhorns, neighbors rallied to her defense – or perhaps, more correctly, to the defense of the integrity of the neighborhood. "One of my neighbors accosted one of the demonstrators – because they had violated our ordinance against picketing. And the police, instead of arresting the demonstrator, arrested the neighbor!"

In spite of the expressions of support that typically come after such picketing, the violation of the privacy of one's home is an enormous strain, especially when young children are involved. Judith Harmon recalled her fear when her two children were of elementary school age. "I never once, not one time ever, let my children go to or from school alone. And I'm only four blocks from the school. Every other student walked without their parent, but my situation was different and I just could not. I was just frightened by the threats, and I just couldn't do it. . . . They [children] hated it."

Ed Lever had teenaged children at the time of his most intense harassment by antiabortionists. "Well, I was used to this kind of thing – because of my civil rights activities, it had happened to me before. I was much more concerned about my children and, believe me, my daughter – the oldest, who is now thirty – really resented me. She knew I was doing what she thought was the right thing to do, but the embarrassment to a kid going to high school! We have talked about it since. She said, 'I knew at the time deep down I was proud of what you were doing, but it was hurting me because I felt I was being singled out instead of you.'"

A number of the men interviewed mentioned the toll their involvement in abortion took on their wives. Zachary Harris attributes the breakup of his marriage in large part to the strain of being constantly harassed by antiabortionists. Although the vast majority of those studied reported the steadfast support of family members, some acknowledged that their spouses had difficulty with abortion – some on practical grounds, some on more ideological grounds. Horace Freeman, after speaking eloquently for some time about women's rights to reproductive freedom, paused and said, "It's interesting . . . my wife has a dichotomy. She believes in everything I just said to you. She just wishes I weren't involved. . . . She worries about people attacking me." Eugene Fox – who is subject to much antiabortion activity – commented of his wife's more ideological objection, "She supports *me*, she doesn't necessarily believe in abortion. We talked about it. She just said, 'I don't think I could ever have one.' And that's the way it should be. You don't have to have an abortion to be a member of the human race."

An identity as an abortion provider affected many other areas of these respondents' lives, especially those who lived in smaller towns. Abortion has become so thoroughly politicized in American culture, one can conclude, that those associated with abortion find they cannot escape the issue even when they become involved in activities that arguably have nothing to do with abortion. The following three examples illustrate how the abortion issue can shadow providers as they attempt, respectively, civic involvement, church affiliation and a private social life.

Bill Swinton, as I have already shown above, made more efforts than most providers to attempt some dialogue with the antiabortionists in his community. Moreover, the nature of his medical practice and the extent of his community activities make him less vulnerable than some to the most negative assumptions about cold-hearted, money-grabbing abortionists. Swinton is a practitioner of family medicine and thus provides more services, to a wider range of community members, than is typical for physicians who specialize in abortion. He and his wife have been extremely active for many years in their church. Perhaps the most unusual feature of Swinton's life, in comparison to others studied for this project, was the fact that in the pre-*Roe* era, he and his wife offered housing and financial assistance to pregnant unwed young women who could not obtain abortions – a practice more commonly advocated by the antiabortion movement. In some respects, then, Swinton is an abortion provider who has achieved a position of considerable respect and devotion in his community. Nevertheless, when he ran for his fourth term on the local school board in the late 1980s, a coordinated campaign by local fundamentalists was able to defeat him – campaigning against him solely on the basis of his provision of abortion.

While about half of those interviewed for this study mentioned belonging to a church or synagogue, Thomas Darrow is distinctive as the only one who claimed to be a fundamentalist Christian. Raised as a Southern Baptist, Darrow had to undergo a period of soul searching to reconcile the conservative views of his church with his belief in the necessity of legal abortion. "I'm a strong believer in the rights of the individual. . . . In the Southern Baptist convention it's called the 'Priesthood of the Believer,' where each individual has the right to live their life the way they see fit after serious consideration, prayer, whatever, then you make your own decision for yourself and you live your life in that manner and you're responsible for it, instead of the Pope telling you you've got to do this or you've got to do that. . . . I've always been a strong believer in individual rights as long as it didn't cause harm. . . . I don't go along with the arguments about the right of the fetus. . . . If you look at it historically, according to ancient Jewish law, abortion was recognized up until the time of quickening, which is about twenty weeks. . . . The other thing is, I've seen the other side of the street, I've seen when elective abortion is not available. I don't want us to go back to that."

But if Darrow has been able to reconcile for himself his religious beliefs and his support of abortion, finding a church in the various communities in which he has lived that was accepting of his job has always been more challenging. Discussing the contrast between two Southern Baptist churches – one in a large city in the South, the other in his present small town – Darrow said,

> The minister [in the large city] came by to visit – I think he brought his wife. . . . I told him, "You understand, we drink." He said, "That's not a problem for me." . . . The Southern Baptist convention has a definite pro-

hibition against consumption and sale of alcohol. I said, "You also understand, I do elective abortions." He said, "That's not a problem for me
either. If it's a problem for you, that's your problem." I felt very comfortable at that church, mainly because one of the prominent local gyns that
was doing therapeutic abortions in the local hospital was a deacon in
the church, so I just fit right in. The same denomination, here in this
town, we joined a very small church when we came up, a lot of strong
antiabortion sentiment in the church, no pro-choice in the church at all
among any of the membership. Some of the members you felt were a little frosty and you wondered if that might not be the reason, but you
never know. We ended up leaving that church, primarily for that reason.

   Well, we finally joined the Presbyterian church. The same thing
came up, same questions, that's not a problem. . . . It seems the Presbyterian church at least addressed it. In our church there is a statement that
as far as the denomination is concerned, elective abortion is a decision
each individual has to make for themselves; the church will not propose
to impose their wishes on the individual, which I thought was kind of
nice.

But though Darrow and his family have found a church that by
and large accepts them and with which they are comfortable, the
abortion issue can occasionally cause awkwardness. "I'm in a Sunday school class with a bunch of old men. There's only one other guy
in there my age – he's a teacher in the high school – we're the only two
guys under sixty. It's an interesting group. . . . These old guys just get
so fired up, they're so emotional, black and white, right and wrong,
and he and I are sitting over there with the wisdom of our youth saying, 'Loosen up, fellows, it really isn't that bad.' . . . We got some strong
antiabortion people in there. One of them was talking about AIDS
and how we're all on our way to hell with all this abortion and homo-
sexuality." When asked if he responded to such remarks, Darrow replied, "Only when there's a gross mistake in the fact. . . . I don't try to
change people's opinions." Speaking more generally about his decision not to confront his fellow church members on abortion, Darrow
said, "I'm prepared to take some heat. . . . I've endured embarrassment and, you know, people making some very unsavory com-

ments, which I assume [was because] people didn't know I was directly involved in it. Otherwise I'd end up hating the people and I don't want to do that. I just disagree with their opinions – I don't hate the people."

Finally, the abortion issue can have an impact on the providers' social lives, as Oswald Watson and his wife, Alice, have found in trying to establish themselves in the community to which they have recently moved. Watson, the semi-retired obstetrician-gynecologist who did not perform abortions until he moved to the West Coast and was trained in abortion procedures, is now employed by a clinic where he performs abortions several days a week. Watson has received a fair number of phone calls in the night and, as mentioned above, is subject to heckling by picketers at his clinic, but he and his wife suggested that it was most difficult settling into a new community with the identity of abortion provider. As Alice Watson said, "It's such a different thing. He came from being a highly regarded physician in the community to something of a pariah. It's just not the same thing. There is just no opportunity to meet other, just regular physicians in the town or anywhere else. There is a strong Catholic group in town. . . . I know of one example when we – we like to play bridge – and these Catholic women wouldn't play with us."

The Watsons related an incident that occurred at a dinner and bridge party at the home of new acquaintances who apparently were very conservative on the abortion issue but knew of Watson's involvement. As he put it, "Bridge players are nuts; they don't care whether they play with the devil, as long as they are good players. We play with these people, salt of the earth types, it's their twenty-fifth anniversary, they invite us for dinner and their daughter is there with three young children. . . . In the course of the conversation at the dinner table, Sandy, the daughter, asks, 'Dr. Watson, what kind of doctor are you?' "

Watson managed to get out, 'I'm a gynecologist,' and at that point in the conversation both Alice Watson and their hostess began to talk loudly over him, making any more of his statement unintelligible, which Watson claims was unnecessary. "I certainly would have told them, but I wouldn't with the three kids at the table." After the children had left the table, however, Watson turned to his hosts' daughter, known to be a born-again Christian, and said, 'Now Sandy, you asked me what I do, and I believe strongly in what I do. I want you to know, I wouldn't permit it not to tell you. I do nothing but abortions.'" Sandy's reaction to this statement, according to Watson, was, "Oh, dear."

Reflecting on how Oswald Watson's new identity as abortion provider affected their status in the community, Alice Watson was both wistful and philosophical. On the one hand, she was very aware of the loss of "a certain place in the community," which they used to enjoy when Watson was simply an obstetrician/gynecologist in private practice. On the other hand, she was well aware of how much greater the strain would be on her if she were still raising young children, and if they were living in a place that was less tolerant than the West Coast. In response to a more general question about her reaction to abortion-related social slights, she answered simply, "It doesn't matter anymore. It would have mattered at one time, but not now." Both Watsons, finally, spoke with evident satisfaction of the strong affirmation of Oswald's abortion practice by their two grown sons.

To summarize, abortion work has the potential to spill over into virtually all aspects of the providers' lives. Never knowing if a professional or a social encounter will provoke antiabortion feelings, abortion providers find themselves maintaining a certain low-level wariness in most of their dealings. However, with respect to the militants who harass them at home and office, the vigilance of abortion providers is of an immediate and practical nature. Physicians hire security consultants, are in regular contact with lawyers apprising them of what actions can be taken against trespassers, become experts in such previous exotica as the antidotes to the butyric acid (an extremely hard-to-eradicate chemical that has the smell of human vomit) that is splashed into their workplaces, carefully examine all suspicious-looking packages sent to them at the office and at home, and, in general, learn that they have reservoirs of strength and tenacity of which they had been unaware. Though there are, of course, variations in both the levels of harassment that different respondents in this study receive, as well as in their psychological capacity to absorb such stress, Ron Ehrlich appeared to speak for most when he described his gradual "desensitization." "The first time, you've never been picketed, and all of a sudden you see pickets, and it shakes you up. And then they come two times, three times, four times, and after a while, it doesn't shake you up anymore. I used to say, 'Well, I don't care if they come to the clinic, as long they don't come into my office.' Then you find out on the next day that they go to your office. So you live through that one. And you say, 'Oh, so let them come to my office. I don't care as long as they don't come to my home.' So they come to your home. And you get anxious . . . and then it gets to the point where you're desensitized. They couldn't do anything to me right now."

SUSTAINING A COMMITMENT TO ABORTION WORK

Given the ambivalent, sometimes overtly hostile, stance toward abortion work on the part of some medical colleagues, and the harassment of the antiabortion movement, how do abortion providers sustain their commitment to this work? Not surprisingly, many among this group experience powerful emotions as a result of their beleaguered situation. In addition to the rage and fear antiabortion forces provoke, abortion providers feel betrayed by a medical community that has marginalized them, and abandoned by both political leaders and a law enforcement system that have – in providers' views – been unconscionably slow to acknowledge the seriousness of the violence of the antiabortion movement. Nonetheless, of all those interviewed who are still in active medical practice (approximately thirty-five), only two physicians no longer provide abortions, confessing to emotional "burnout" (though each still strongly supports legal abortion). The simplest answer – and ultimately the most compelling one – as to what sustains the others is their unwavering belief in the necessity of what they are doing. Ken Gordon expressed a common sentiment when he said, "If I never had to do another abortion again, I wouldn't miss it. People say, 'Oh, you do it for the money.' Money be damned! I get five times as much for doing a delivery. [Performing abortions] gives me no pleasure. The only positive thing about it is that I know it's being done by a trained physician, under sterile conditions, in a safe facility – so the patient is not going to bleed to death, get infected, or have much pain . . . and I never want to see us go back to those old, not good days." But if such a conviction is the bottom line for all these abortion providers, we can still point to some interesting variations in the strategies used to make this often stressful work more tenable.

David Bennett is the most striking example of a practitioner who has found in abortion work enormous opportunities for creativity and professional growth. As discussed in chapter 4, Bennett, who had done many illegal abortions, early on became committed to making the abortion experience as "humanistic" as possible, devoting much of his attention to pain management. After *Roe*, Bennett went into "retreat" for a period of time, to recover from the stress caused by several years of full-time illegal abortion work. When he reemerged, he found himself drawn back – to his surprise – to abortion provision, rather than to the more general family practice for which he originally trained. "It became my professional work. I devoted my best effort to improving procedures and techniques, ways of providing service to make it as good and humane as my abilities would allow. So all along I kept observing, and I'm a good observer, . . . and I've learned from the women what happens when I do this and when I do that. . . . I'm not simply going to be an extension of that machine, just mechanical. . . . Every woman that comes through is different. Every experience is different. Her counseling is different, her pain management may be different, they way you interact with her is different. With one, you may tell jokes, with one you tell stories, with another you cry – what she brings and interacts with you is different."

The founding of the National Abortion Federation (NAF) in 1976, a group composed of physicians and others involved in abortion provision, was a particularly significant event for Bennett, as he met others who shared his deep interest in the broader aspects of abortion services. Speaking of the atmosphere of the early NAF gatherings, Bennett said, "There were some big issues to work on. . . . The positions people held [on standards for abortion services] were slowly changing . . . so I began to deal more on 'quality of abortion care,' the pain management program, counseling, how to do training. I began to work with Anna [his future wife], a really good trainer, and I learned so much from her. It began a work that we could do together with her knowledge of psychology and training. We worked together very well in developing a unified program."

Over the years Bennett has also drawn tremendous gratification from teaching abortion techniques, something he frequently does at workshops organized by NAF. But the most fundamental source of gratification for him remains the abortion procedure itself. Bennett several times referred to his medicine as "artwork." This "artistry" encompasses not only making the operation as physically painless as possible, but also treating the patient with sufficient dignity and concern so that her abortion experience might serve as a springboard to a higher degree of self-awareness and esteem. This focus on the total patient, in Bennett's words, "has been a sustaining element, which has kept it [abortion work] from being boring and repetitious."

Bennett's preoccupation with the totality of the "abortion experience" is somewhat unusual. But, as Ethan Stevenson did at Preterm, many providers feel it is important to have some interaction with the abortion patient beyond the procedure itself–finding this of benefit to themselves as well as to her. It is obviously easier for those who operate their own clinics or provide abortions in their own offices to do so than for those who are employed and supervised by others. As an example, we can contrast the responses of Eugene Fox, who worked for a time in a for-profit clinic, managed by others, to those of Marty Kaufman, who does abortions in his own office. Speaking of abortion "entrepreneurs" who emerged shortly after *Roe*, Fox said, "They would put up these clinics and then they would bring in doctors, and the game was, how many can you do in an afternoon? There was a lot of pressure and a lot of anxiety and none of us liked the way we had to practice. You didn't get a chance to know the patients ahead of time. . . . We were like cogs in the wheel."[13] Kaufman, who performs abortions both at a clinic he operates and in his private practice, describes his reactions in these terms. "At the clinic, I take what is given to me. I always talk with the patient, saying, 'I am Dr. Kaufman' . . . but I'm really dependent on the counselor for the support and nurturing. In my office I'm dependent on myself. . . . The difference is that I know the patient much better than I do in the clinic setting. It's a much more complete process for me, taking the patient from the beginning through the whole thing. I set out a block of time of an hour and a half per patient. That is exorbitant as far as the time investment . . . but I enjoy that. And that's important for me. If I would turn it into more of a treadmill, then I would lose that gratification."

Others suggested that their political involvement in the broader pro-choice movement was a stimulating and energizing activity that was both an outgrowth of their actual abortion work and in turn helped to sustain it. Caleb Barrington, for example, relished the memory of participating in one of the major abortion cases that ultimately reached the Supreme Court, in which he helped find patients to offer depositions and he himself served as an expert witness. A number of those interviewed periodically testify before Congress and in state legislatures on abortion-related matters, just as they used to do before *Roe.*

Predictably, interaction with other providers is a major source of support and affirmation and helps sustain this group's commitment to abortion practice. Formally, this interaction happens at several organizations, such as NAF and the Association of Reproductive Health Professionals. Contrasting the colleagueship that typifies NAF meetings with the coldness that he experiences from many in his local medical community, David Bennett said, "I go to NAF, people say nice things about you, they respect me and other people in this field. . . . There you can go and be acknowledged for the contribution you have made, for the work you have done." Daniel Fieldstone too drew a contrast between the camaraderie he experienced at NAF and the lukewarm support given many abortion providers at the most relevant mainstream organization, the American College of Obstetricians and Gynecologists. As he put it, "The people at NAF are like family to me."

On a more informal level, nearly all of those interviewed spoke of the importance of having other abortion providers as colleagues with whom they could routinely share concerns. Of course, abortion providers are not unique among medical professionals in seeking out formal and informal ties with colleagues. The special circumstances facing this group, however, give their efforts at community building a special valence. This group depends on colleagues not only to share the latest techniques, or to give the professional affirmation that mainstream medicine withholds, but also for support in the face of antiabortion attacks. Such support ranges from the practical–how to deal, legally, in the office and clinic settings with picketing and blockades, how to choose among the latest technologies for personal and workplace security–to the more emotional–how to remain committed to an activity that is so socially explosive.

But if some providers manage to find in abortion work a source of creativity, and nearly all of the others remain because of a profound political commitment, the fact remains that, for most, abortion work *per se* is not particularly gratifying, both because of its technically un-challenging nature and the professional opportunities missed be-cause of its demands. Louise Thomas, one of the very few providers in her remote New England location, spoke with particular poi-gnancy to this point when she said, "I feel I'm wasting my career. I was trained as an ob/gyn specialist, and I'm spending too much time fighting rearguard actions in a battle that is essentially won, because it's time in history for this [legal abortion] to happen. But the fact is that there is still opposition and it's taking up my energy . . . and yet, other people aren't [involved]. . . . and so, here I am." Similarly, Mir-iam Harkin, whose abortion practice over the years grew to the point that she had to forego obstetrics, spoke with wistfulness of the trade-off she had felt compelled to make. "Obstetrics was very gratifying. I really enjoyed it. . . . I realize that abortion is an opportunity for a woman to get a second run on a bad life, but it's not the most gratify-ing part of my practice; procedurally it's so routine." Eugene Fox, fi-nally, gave a strong statement of the conflict some providers, espe-cially those trained as ob/gyns, felt between abortion work and other aspects of their professional lives. "I like obstetrics, I like delivering babies and talking to patients about their expectations. . . . I really don't like to do abortions. The act of abortion really goes against my own personal feelings about obstetrics. I have spent an awful lot of time trying to save babies and prevent prematurity . . . so abortion doesn't really fit my feelings–but on the other hand, that is not what I am here for, and I would rather see them done properly than to pick up the pieces after. That is totally unnecessary. I look at the need for abortion as a failure on our part to impart the proper information to young women. We are just not getting the right message to a large number of women soon enough to prevent the unwanted pregnancy."

Thus, the experiences of this group suggest that those who were seemingly most satisfied with abortion provision were those in a position to integrate it with other professional activities. Such integration not only permits time to do other, more professionally challenging activities, but also can confer the legitimacy among medical colleagues and the general public that the full-time abortion provider often lacks. Ron Ehrlich, who is the director of both a freestanding abortion clinic and a freestanding birth center, administers a department in his large suburban hospital, and is a senior partner in a busy private practice, perceives his professional status in these terms: "I've got nurses today that are staunch Catholics who work in that hospital and they hate me for [performing abortions], but they still respect me for everything else I do. So it [the range of activities] has carried me. I maintain a very high, I think, quality of practice, and a very high concern for people, and I've shown it. . . . I have gotten involved in a lot of things . . . and I don't let what they [abortion opponents] are going to say stop me."

The experiences of this group seem to demonstrate, therefore, that the abortion delivery system that has evolved in the United States since *Roe*– in which a relatively small number of physicians perform the majority of all abortions – may have advantages for the patient (it is highly desirable, after all, to have one's abortion performed by someone who has done thousands of such procedures) but is far from ideal for the physician, given the drawbacks of full-time abortion work.

THE NECESSITY OF ABORTION, THE LIMITATIONS OF ABORTION

By definition, all the physicians who appear in this book are "prochoice," but that vague phrase of course covers a range of feelings about abortion and about their own roles as abortion providers. In some respects, the physicians in this group have quite disparate attitudes toward abortion. For some in this group, and for other Americans who consider themselves pro-choice, abortion is "sad but necessary," as Simon Ross expressed it; while for others, a woman's decision to have an abortion can be seen as a positive first step in taking control of her life. For a number of those interviewed, overcoming early religious training, which taught the immorality of abortion, was necessary psychologically to be able to perform abortions. Yet for the most currently devout person in this group, Thomas Darrow, his strong sense of a personal relationship with Jesus Christ – and especially his identification with Christ's nonconformity – is precisely what enables him to do abortion work. "When I felt the world was going against me, or perhaps I should try to go with the flow a bit more, as a Christian, as a follower of Jesus Christ, I started studying his life and really Jesus Christ did *not* go with the flow. Here's a guy that was raised in a Jewish family and very knowledgeable about Jewish literature and on his way to being a rabbi, actually was a rabbi, and all of a sudden makes a sharp 180-degree turn and says, 'Wait a minute, folks, this isn't the way to do it.' . . . Talk about taking heat! Let's get real! So when I think about that, it [decision to provide abortions] almost becomes a religious experience, it really does."

For some, the belief in the necessity of abortion is grounded in "humanism," or more specifically, the imperative to practice humanistic medicine. Others more explicitly use the language of feminism to defend abortion. Predictably, such sentiments were voiced very strongly by some of the women interviewed, especially those who had themselves undergone abortions in the pre-*Roe* era, but some of the most impassioned feminist statements came from male respondents. Paul Temple said, "It comes down to who is the patient. Is the woman the patient, or is the fetus the patient? One or the other is the patient. I've never heard a fetus talk to me. I've heard thousands and thousands of women share their pain, their desperation, and their hopelessness . . . especially with the younger patients that come to us, twelve or fourteen years old – their life expectancy may be eighty-four years! . . . We're not talking about five- or ten-year survival rates, or remission of cancer . . . we're talking about the opportunity to help them change the rest of their lives for seventy years."

Bob Phillips, a crusty ex-Marine, spoke of his worries about the complacency in the pro-choice movement in these terms. "The men stink, forget about them, they are useless. I mean, they enjoy their little efforts and their problem is ended. They came and went, in essence, and it's still a woman's problem. It *shouldn't* be a woman's problem but it *is* a woman's problem in today's society, and the women are going to have to stay tuned to what the antiabortionists are doing."

For some, the overriding consideration in their stand on abortion is the realization that their own philosophical views, whatever they are, should be subordinated to those of the only one whose decision it is to make – the pregnant woman. Rosalind Greene reflected on her practice shortly after the *Roe* decision. "I was the only one doing obstetrics in my area, and I began to see more of the desperate women out seeking abortions. And the more I listened to what they had to say about their reasons, the more convinced I was that I should not make the decision. It was not a medical decision, by and large; it was more in knowing what she could and could not live with in her life." Ken Gordon spoke similarly, reminiscing about a patient "who came in and out of the hospital nine times. She just couldn't make up her mind about an abortion. Eventually she carried to term. I just find it impossible to put myself in other people's shoes." Though this view of the pregnant woman as ultimate decision-maker was by and large shared by nearly all interviewed, others were more willing to voice some judgments on the reasons women sought abortions. Some expressed their disappointment at repeat abortions, and several physicians explicitly stated – speaking hypothetically – that they would not perform an abortion on the basis of the sex of the fetus.

In some respects, then, the diverse responses to abortion among this group mirror a similar range of attitudes among the pro-choice public, who support abortion from a variety of standpoints. Yet the particular circumstances of this provider group, who deal with abortion on a daily basis, provide them with a unique perspective on both the necessity and, ultimately, the limitations of legal abortion. Just as I have argued that in the pre-*Roe* era, this group was in a privileged position to see the results of illegal abortion, so these providers now, some twenty plus years after legalization, can uniquely appreciate the combination of human frailty, imperfect contraceptive technology, and the workings of fate that will always make some abortion inevitable.

For these providers, one ironic but telling indication of the inevitability of abortion – no matter how hotly it is politically contested – is the steady stream of avowed antiabortionists who turn up as patients. As Bob Phillips said, with a mixture of disgust and bemusement, "The same old thing, the double standards. We have antiabortionists who have waved banners downtown come in for their daughters or themselves. We've had nuns who have abortions. We have nurses that refuse to take care of salines[14] come in and have abortions." Charles Swensen was startled to recognize in his procedure room, accompanying her daughter for an abortion, an antiabortion leader whom he had recently debated. The conversation that Morris Fischer had with an antiabortion activist who sought an abortion for her daughter helps us understand why abortion providers develop a more complex view of abortion (and perhaps of human nature) than others less directly involved. "We had a woman come in here. Admittedly, she was very honest. She said, 'I'm a member of the River Prolife Council, but when it touches your own home, you have to forget the philosophy. You have to do what you have to do.' But she told me that she will still go out on the picket line."[15]

But if these abortion-providing physicians see safe and legal abortion as both necessary and inevitable, they also are troubled by the volume of abortion in the contemporary United States. These physicians, who in some cases literally risk their lives to provide abortions, most emphatically do not see legal abortion as a sufficient condition, in itself, of "reproductive freedom." Indeed, one of the greatest frustrations that this group expresses is that the fight to protect legal abortion, which has preoccupied them and their allies since 1973, has distracted their attention from the effort to win political acceptance of a genuine program of reproductive health. Such a program would encompass a broad expansion of sex education efforts, prenatal services, contraceptive services (including far more research than is currently the case),[16] as well as the availability of abortion. Daniel

Fieldstone's words mostly convey the disappointment felt at the present status of reproductive health in the United States, but also suggest the different future he and his colleagues would like to help construct:

> Our generation has been trying to pass the torch to the next one to show that there has never been a time when the termination of pregnancy didn't take place. And there's no society where it doesn't take place. What one determines is the circumstances, how it takes place and whether it takes place in a medically safe and humane environment or is criminalized – that's what we try to make people think about. But over and above that, if we weren't such a hypocritical society, we would be educating our young people to understand the limitations, uses, abuses of sex. And the relationship between sex and love, and the necessity to understand and selectively control reproduction, so that they can have a productive and meaningful adult life. If this were a rational society, we'd have fewer unintended pregnancies and far fewer abortions. . . . It's insane that 54 percent of our pregnancies are unintended.[17]

CHAPTER SEVEN

Assuring a Future for Legal Abortion

Despite the difficulties associated with abortion provision, all but two of the forty-five physicians interviewed for this book remained committed to this work throughout their careers. The common factor binding this otherwise disparate group was their experience, as young physicians, of witnessing the effects of illegal abortion. Now, however, as this group and others in the first generation of legal abortion providers near retirement, a number of questions are raised with increasing urgency in the pro-choice movement. Who will replace this "conscience" generation? What will motivate younger physicians and contemporary medical students, who have never had the pre-*Roe* emergency room experiences of the older group, to do this work? And will medical institutions offer adequate training in abortion techniques in order to assure a continuity of this service?

These questions are raised at a moment of unusual ferment not only within the field of abortion politics, but within the broader field of health politics as a whole, as the country wrestles with the issue of health care reform. Unresolved legal issues pertaining to restrictions on abortion, the societal response to antiabortion violence, the eventual status of RU-486 (the "abortion pill"), and the outcome of the health reform debate – all will affect the future of abortion services in the United States.[1] This chapter will describe some of these larger issues, whose eventual resolution will have an impact on abortion provision, and will examine the unique role that the medical community might play in addressing the crisis in abortion services.

THE LEGAL CLIMATE

Although in 1992 the Supreme Court, in the *Planned Parenthood v. Casey* decision, upheld the central holding of *Roe v. Wade* – that there is a constitutional right to an abortion before viability – the *Casey* decision permits extensive regulation of abortion services. In legal terms, one of the most significant aspects of that decision is the shift from "strict scrutiny" to the lesser standard of "undue burden" with respect to restrictions that can be put on abortion. In practical terms, this means that it is now far easier for antiabortion forces to impede efforts to provide and to obtain abortions.

Some of the more recently imposed restrictions have the most severe impact on women seeking abortions, for example the various parental notification and consent requirements for teenagers. While research suggests that most teenagers who have abortions do, in fact, tell their parents, for the minority who do not, often young women from troubled families, such requirements have been shown to be highly problematic.[2] The mandated twenty-four- or forty-eight-hour delays now in place in a number of states most significantly affect rural women, who often have to travel long distances to reach an abortion provider. A lawyer involved in a suit against such a mandated delay requirement in South Dakota gives a sense of the impact of these delays on those seeking abortions:

> In that state – one of the poorest in the country – there is only one abortion provider, Dr. Buck Williams in Sioux Falls. A recently enacted law requires that a woman be provided certain state-mandated information a minimum of 24 hours before her abortion. The information must be provided by the physician who will perform the abortion.
>
> Because South Dakota is a large rural state, 36 percent of Dr. Williams's patients who received abortions in 1991 traveled 200 or more miles round trip. Nearly half of those traveled 600 or more miles round trip, six to eight hours each way. Many of them work at low-wage jobs, where they are paid at hourly rates with no sick leave. The day's trip means losing a day's pay. The 24 hour waiting period means another day of lost wages and the need for a second trip – often on snowy and icy roads – or the cost of an overnight stay, in addition to the cost of child

care (assuming it can be arranged). The need to be away from job and home for two days also compromises the woman's ability to keep her abortion confidential.[3]

Other recently upheld restrictions have significant implications for the provider, as well as the patient. Chief among these are the mandated counseling provisions now in place in a number of states. In some of these cases, the physician providing the abortion or making the referral – as opposed to other clinic or office staff – is obliged to deliver to the patient a scripted message about such matters as all the risks of the abortion procedure, fetal development, fetal pain, and the social services available to those who choose to carry their pregnancies to term. While it is true, as I have argued in this book, that many abortion providers actually express a wish for more contact with the abortion recipient, the delivery of a prewritten script is a mockery of genuine abortion counseling.[4] Such mandated counseling requirements have the net effect of burdening the physician's schedule, delaying the abortion for the patient, and making it even less likely that she will receive authentic counseling.

But perhaps the most consequential of all these proposed restrictions, from the providers' standpoint, is the strict – and extremely vague – language regulating later abortions. In Utah, for example, in the aftermath of *Casey*, a judge upheld a prohibition on post-twenty-week abortions, except those necessary to save a woman's life, prevent "grave" damage to her health, or prevent the birth of a child with "grave" defects."[5] This law, and others like it, are of enormous concern to providers because of the unclarified, highly subjective nature of the language used. As the participants in this study found out when they attempted to offer committee-approved abortions in the pre-*Roe* era, there are profound differences among physicians as to what constitutes a "threat" to a woman's life, "grave" damage to her health, and so on. In essence, statutes such as the one described above could well recreate the "gray area" abortions and legal precariousness of the pre-*Roe* era. A key difference, however, between the pre-*Roe* period and the present is that there is now in place a network of anti-abortion activists – within both the medical and legal communities – that presumably will be far more aggressive in challenging gray area abortions than was the case in the past. It thus seems inevitable that in states that adopt statutes similar to the one in Utah, the number of providers willing to perform later abortions will diminish even more. It is true that most abortions in the United States take place within the first trimester of pregnancy; nevertheless, even though fewer than 1 percent of all abortions in the United States in 1988 were performed after twenty weeks, that figure still represents more than ten thousand procedures.[6] It is also the case, ironically, that the restrictions mentioned above–mandated waiting periods and especially parental notification regulations–may themselves *result in* later abortions, because of the impediments they pose to those seeking abortions. In Mississippi, for example, there was an approximate 20 percent increase in second trimester abortions after the state imposed a mandatory waiting period, forcing many in that rural state to make two separate visits to a clinic.[7] Thus, we can anticipate that it will be more difficult for those who might need later abortions in the near future to find them.

The most likely legal scenario in the aftermath of *Casey* is that abortion regulation will vary considerably from state to state. These variations in turn may further intensify the "regionalization" of abortion services, a phenomenon already evident in the mid-1990s, when abortion services are found in only 16 percent of U.S. counties and there are only a handful of providers in the country who perform late-term (post-twenty-four week) abortions. Such regionalization of course is also reminiscent of the years immediately preceding *Roe*, in which women traveled to "liberal" states which had already legalized abortion. While *Casey* stipulates that no state can ban abortions outright, both the number of restrictions imposed on provider and patient and the perceptions of how aggressively local authorities will be in monitoring such restrictions will help determine whether a given location will have abortion services. Furthermore, the availability of abortions, especially later ones, is not only dependent on an individual physician's willingness to provide the service; the various factors mentioned above will have a chilling effect on *hospitals'* receptivity to abortion services. Women who become sick or discover fetal anomalies late in pregnancies will be especially hard pressed to find hospitals that permit later abortions.

VIOLENCE AND ABORTION PROVISION

There is no adequate way of quantifying the effect of the antiabortion movement on the willingness of physicians to provide abortion. As I have argued, it would be a mistake to overestimate the influence of antiabortionists in explaining the provider shortage, and thereby to overlook other factors, such as the long-standing ambivalence of the medical establishment toward abortion. At the same time, it would be absurd to deny that antiabortion harassment has a chilling effect on abortion provision, especially when it becomes violent. Some providers leave the field; other younger doctors doubtless decide never to even become involved with abortion. Any speculation, therefore, about the future availability of abortion must take into account society's likely responses to such violence, as well as intensifying splits within the antiabortion movement about the wisdom of such tactics.

Clearly, the murders in 1993 and 1994 of five individuals within the abortion-providing community were critical turning points in the public's toleration of antiabortion terrorism, causing both an outcry against it and a demand for more protection of abortion facilities. In sharp contrast to the presidential administrations of Ronald Reagan and George Bush, President Clinton and his attorney general, Janet Reno, forcefully condemned such violence and pledged to find appropriate governmental responses to the problem of protecting abortion facilities. The murder of David Gunn, a physician, gave impetus to a bill that was already in process in both houses of Congress, the FACE legislation (Freedom of Access to Clinic Entrance). This bill, which designates blockades and other disruptive actions at clinic sites to be federal offenses and imposes substantial penalties for such activities, was approved by Congress in late 1993 and signed by President Clinton in 1994. In response to the murders of John Britton, a physician, and James Barrett, his volunteer escort, in the summer of 1994, Reno dispatched federal marshals to offer round-the-clock protection to those clinics across the country deemed most at risk of violence – a step long called for by the pro-choice movement. In another step long urged by providers, the FBI announced an inquiry to see if a conspiracy existed among networks of antiabortion terrorists. Also, in the wake of the escalation of violence against providers, a

number of states and localities have passed "antistalking" legislation, which attempts to limit the harassment of individual providers
both at their homes and elsewhere. Similarly motivated by antiabortion tactics – in this case, the tracking down and harassment of clinic
patients and staff through their license plate numbers – a portion of
the Omnibus Crime Bill of 1994 contained a provision making it illegal for state motor vehicle agencies to release identifying information
to the public. Finally, a 1994 Supreme Court case, *Madsen v. Women's
Health Services*, established the legality of a thirty-six-foot buffer
zone around clinics and the use of noise restrictions.[8]

The Gunn-Britton-Barrett murders, followed shortly thereafter
by those of Shannon Lowney and Leanne Nichols, receptionists in
two Massachusetts clinics, and clinic firebombings, have also accen-
tuated splits within the antiabortion movement. In a pattern quite
predictable to students of social movements, the more mainstream
wing of the antiabortion movement, e.g., the National Right to Life
Committee and the National Conference of Catholic Bishops, has unequivocally condemned such violence, while the more extremist segments of the movement have not.[9] Many in the more mainstream
wing of the movement not only feel genuine repugnance at the terrorism associated with the radical wing, they also oppose such activity because it erodes public support for the antiabortion movement as
a whole. For those in the more extremist groups, on the other hand,
widespread "public support" is increasingly beside the point.

During the Reagan-Bush years, at the height of the political
strength of the mainstream antiabortion movement – when its leaders were welcomed at the White House – the moderates arguably held
some sway over more militant factions. At the present moment, with
their political clout significantly diminished, the mainstream organizations seem less capable than ever of controlling the violent tendencies of other groups. Thus, some antiabortion groups, in the aftermath of the 1992 election, seem to be conforming to the classic pattern
of a social movement increasingly turning to violence when it perceives it has little chance in the conventional political arena.

Taken together, the above-mentioned trends point to a future in
which there may be a reduction in the overall number of disruptions
of abortion services, but there will continue to be occasional acts of

extreme violence. The forceful response of local police to attempted blockades and sieges of clinics – already evident in the summer of 1993 in the immediate aftermath of the Gunn killing – and the willingness of judges in some localities to impose more severe fines and jail sentences has already resulted in a downward trend in such incidents. Yet firebombings of abortion clinics in 1993 and 1994 – the act of only one person or a small group – increased at the same time that such large-scale blockades were decreasing.[10]

While there have been, in the mid-1990s, encouraging signs of official determination to combat antiabortion violence, the future course of both this violence and government's response is difficult to predict. (Governmental response of course depends on the particular presidential administration in office; in contrast to the Clinton administration's support of FACE and the dispatching of federal marshals to protect clinics, the Bush administration only a few years earlier went to court on behalf of Operation Rescue in a Supreme Court case concerning harassment of clinic employees and patients.)[11]

Moreover, even should violence at clinics diminish, abortion providers in the 1990s are facing an unprecedented round of aggressive legal action against them by antiabortion groups. Law firms have been formed which specialize in abortion malpractice. Antiabortion groups have compiled lists of physicians and other health care personnel willing to testify as expert witnesses against providers, and innovative marketing techniques – ranging from television commercials to leafleting outside clinics – are used to recruit women willing to participate in lawsuits against abortion providers.[12] "I'm more afraid of being sued out of business than I am of being shot," one Southern physician told me.

Because of the ongoing vulnerabilities, physical and legal, of abortion provision at the clinic site, many in the pro-choice movement have pinned great hopes on other modes of delivering abortion, a point to which I now turn.

MEDICAL ABORTION

The major alternative at present to surgical abortion is RU-486, the "abortion pill." RU-486 (mifepristone) is an antiprogestin which, used in combination with a prostaglandin, is capable of terminating an early pregnancy (up to eight or nine weeks). The pill, developed by a group of French scientists and popularized by Etienne Baulieu, was approved for use by the French government in 1988. Beyond its use for pregnancy termination, RU-486 also has promising implications for the treatment of certain types of breast cancer, Cushing's Syndrome, glaucoma, and meningiomas. Early studies have also suggested the drug's potential as a contraceptive method and as a postcoital drug that would prevent implantation.[13]

Predictably, since its initial discovery, RU-486 has been continuously embroiled in abortion politics. The drug's availability in France came only after a prolonged process, in which RU-486 was initially approved by the French government; withdrawn from the market one month later by the manufacturer, Roussel-Uclaf, in response to threats of a boycott, primarily by U.S. antiabortionists; and then, two days later – after much public outcry – ordered to be redistributed by the French government, which owns 36 percent of Roussel-Uclaf. In a famous statement calling for redistribution, the French minister of health referred to RU-486 as "the moral property of women."[14]

The political wrangling over RU-486 in the United States has been equally intense. During the administration of George Bush, an FDA ban was imposed on the importation of RU-486 into the United States. This ban was technically for personal use of the drug but had the effect of impeding most scientific research as well. The ban enraged not only the pro-choice community, but the larger medical community as well, who argued that promising medical research was being held hostage to abortion politics. Early on in the Clinton administration, the president expressed his hope that RU-486 would soon be available for use in the United States. Nonetheless, the French manufacturer and its parent company, the German firm Hoechst AG, proceeded with great caution, reflecting their fear of an antiabortion boycott of other Hoechst products, as well as the fear of malpractice suits which might result from use of the new drug. Ultimately, however, in response to pressure from the Clinton administration, Roussel-Uclaf took the quite unusual step of handing over the pill's patent (in the United States) and technology, free of charge, to the Population Council, a nonprofit private research group based in New York. The Council began trials of this drug in a number of sites across the country in late 1994, and the drug is currently expected to be made available to U.S. women sometime in 1996.[15]

Assuming that this nonsurgical method of abortion will eventually become available in the United States, what implications can we anticipate for the delivery of abortion services? A major promise of RU-486 is that abortion provision could be diffused throughout the health care system to a far greater degree than at present, with many more abortions taking place in the privacy of a physician's office. The training necessary to adequately supervise an abortion by this method is less than that required to perform a surgical abortion, and thus one can anticipate a far wider range of physicians offering abortions, including both ob/gyns and primary care providers, as well as, possibly, "midlevel" practitioners (physician assistants, nurse practitioners). In a survey done in 1992 in California of fifteen hundred ob/gyns, 22 percent of those not currently performing abortions said they would prescribe RU-486 if it were legal.[16] If, as RU-486 proponents envision, abortions were taking place "everywhere" in the health care system, and decreasingly in specialized clinics, antiabortionists would have much greater difficulty targeting abortion facilities. Thus both patient and provider would be spared the trauma of militant protests.

For some providers, moreover, medical abortion, as represented by RU-486, may be attractive for reasons that go beyond simply avoiding protestors. This possibility was first suggested to me at a national conference on RU-486 held in 1991. A young female physician, who for several years has been providing abortions at a clinic in the Pacific Northwest, rose from the audience during a discussion period and began to speak of the different nature of the surgical abortions she performed and what she imagined would be the case with medical abortions. She contrasted the passivity of the patient in the former situation, who was having an abortion "done" to her, to the active role the patient took in the latter. "I like that – that the abortion is in her hands, that she is taking that pill." Not having done a follow-up interview with the speaker, I do not know if her comments reflect a genuine ambivalence on her part about performing abortions or simply such fatigue at being the prime target of antiabortionists that she was understandably eager to have others implicated in the act as well. And until RU-486 is more widely available, we will not have a sound research base to compare either providers' or recipients' experiences of the two methods. The speaker's comments, nonetheless, suggest that medical abortion will be a preferable way for some health professionals to provide abortions.

However, several caveats are in order to temper the notion of RU-486 as a "solution" to the abortion problem. First, given that this drug is effective only for early abortions, there will still remain the need for surgical abortions after eight or nine weeks of pregnancy, currently some 50 percent of all abortions in the United States.[17] Moreover, a small percentage–about 4 percent according to some experts–of those receiving RU-486 will not completely abort and will need surgical abortions to complete the procedure. Those who will still perform surgical abortions–especially if in freestanding clinics–may find themselves even more vulnerable to antiabortion attention, as the providers of RU-486 prove difficult to target. Second, some have raised safety concerns at the prospect of physicians in a variety of fields supervising this new form of abortion. Some specialists in obstetrics and gynecology, for example, raise questions about the ability of nonspecialists to adequately diagnose the length of a pregnancy, to assure that the abortion has been completed, and to manage any complications. Third, some within the abortion providing community, while acknowledging the immense advantage of avoiding protestors that RU-486 will make possible, also point to what will be lost with decreased reliance on the clinic model. Especially unfortunate, in this view, will be the loss of the specialized abortion counseling that has long been part of the freestanding clinic movement. The counseling protocols developed in the clinics were designed to help a woman with her decision and to ensure that she is not seeking an abortion because of coercion from a partner or parent. Moreover, considerable efforts are made in many clinics to offer patients in-depth discussions of birth control usage. Many of the private physicians who might be offering RU-486, one can speculate, have neither the training in such counseling nor the time to engage in such "extras." Another complicating aspect of the scenario of abortion provision moving away from clinics and taking place increasingly in private offices is the question of what would become of the thousands of poor and noninsured women who are currently served in the clinics. We can reasonably assume that only those women who have a private physician to begin with will be able to obtain an in-office RU-486 abortion from that provider. This question of the accessibility of RU-486 to impoverished women is of course connected to the larger issue of health reform, but since the poor are highly represented in the population of abortion recipients, we can assume that clinics will always be needed to meet their needs.

Finally, it is not known at this time whether U.S. women will in fact prefer an RU-486-induced abortion to surgical abortion. It is true that in France, where this drug has been available since 1988, a majority of those who were eligible have chosen this option. But outpatient clinic abortions are not available in France, and thus the alternative to RU-486 is hospitalization and an abortion under general anesthesia. In the United States, faced with a choice of having one's abortion and in-clinic recovery period completed within several hours, or having to make a second visit to an office for the subsequent prostaglandin dose, after the original ingestion of RU-486, as the abortion takes place over a period of several days, with somewhat more bleeding than is typical of a surgical abortion, some women (especially those who live at some distance from their abortion provider) will doubtless prefer surgical abortion, even if that means confronting protestors.

A similar form of medical abortion—the use of the drug methotrexate, in combination with another drug, misoprostol—is gradually starting to become available in the United States. Although this combination works similarly to the RU-486 regime as an abortafacient, a significant difference is that both of the drugs in this latter case are already approved for use in the United States. (Though this approval is for uses other than abortion, these drugs can nonetheless be legally dispensed by physicians.) The first clinical trials of this drug combination specifically for the purposes of abortion have reported early success in a small group of patients. But as clinical trials continue, this method received much visibility – and a startled reaction from many in the medical community – when a New York physician went public with a report in the fall of 1994 that he had administered this drug combination to one hundred and twenty-six women, one hundred and twenty-one of whom successfully aborted, with five requiring surgical abortions to complete the process.[18] An unknown number of other physicians are believed to be more quietly dispensing this drug regime as a method of abortion.

While the methotrexate/misoprostol regime poses some of the same limitations as RU-486, these two forms of medical abortion hold such promise for increasing the availability of abortion in areas without clinics, for infusing abortion services into mainstream medical settings, and for their potential other uses, that the pro-choice community is highly committed to making them available in the United States.

HEALTH CARE REFORM

As of this writing, in the immediate aftermath of the spectacular failure of health care legislation in the 1994 Congress – legislation which originally sought to guarantee health care for all Americans – the relation between health reform in the United States and abortion provision remains unclear. Two key lessons that emerged from this first round of health reform politics are, first, that future attempts in this area will undoubtedly be more incremental, rather than the bold remaking of the health care system originally sought in the 1994 Clinton proposal, and, second, and not unexpectedly, that the abortion issue itself has the potential to derail whatever compromise on health care reform is reached in Congress. Periodically, throughout the 1994 debate on health reform, blocs of politicians on both sides of the abortion issue announced their determination not to yield on the issue of abortion coverage.

The initial hopes of the pro-choice movement that such new legislation would mandate universal access to abortion, therefore, have dimmed considerably. Since Clinton's election in 1992, pro-choice forces have been soundly defeated in their attempts to overturn the

Hyde Amendment, which prohibits use of federal funds to pay for abortions of poor women, except in very limited circumstances. These defeats seem to confirm the notion that while the American public is largely supportive of legal abortion, there is considerable reluctance to use tax dollars for subsidized abortions. Thus, one likely scenario for abortion under future health reform is a continuation of the present system, in which some insurance plans cover abortion services and others do not.[19]

But even if eventual health reform does not mandate abortion coverage, forthcoming changes in health care delivery, and especially the move toward "managed care" (in which a "primary provider," usually a family practice physician, serves as gatekeeper to more specialized services), will very likely affect abortion services in several ways. First, given the enormous pressures on cost containment that will accompany any health care reorganization, the freestanding clinic will most likely remain as the major setting for abortion services. Health plans that will cover abortion will in most cases find the most attractive option to be a subcontract with a freestanding clinic for abortion services – as opposed to hospital-based services – simply because the former is the most cost-effective way to deliver abortions.

This cost-driven reliance on clinics for abortion services by newly configured health plans may work somewhat against the efforts to reintegrate abortion into mainstream health care. While, as I have argued, the freestanding clinic is itself a proud creation of the pro-choice community, and no one calls for the abolition of these facilities, there are many abortion providers who feel that the existence of the clinics has, inadvertently, contributed to the marginalization of abortion practice. These providers therefore feel that only if abortion services are delivered throughout the health care system – taking place in hospital outpatient clinics and in doctors' offices as well as in freestanding clinics – will abortion practice overcome its present isolation.

The scenario of newly reorganized health plans relying on clinics for abortion services does not, however, tell us what will happen in those parts of the country that are presently without any abortion providers. In such cases, there indeed might be pressure on local hospitals to establish abortion services. Similarly, some providers might perceive new incentives to establish clinics in those locations. A third alternative – least attractive from the point of view of women needing abortions – is that the health plan in question will reimburse for an abortion from the nearest approved abortion clinic, even if that facility is a day's drive away.[20]

The prospect of abortion services being handled through managed care programs has caused some concern among abortion providers about issues of confidentiality and privacy, which are longstanding staples of abortion provision. Abortion providers argue that some of their patients will want their abortions kept confidential, an option that, of course, will be jeopardized if a referral to an abortion facility must be obtained from one's primary provider. Therefore, these abortion providers call for health plans to make provisions for women to self-refer for abortions.[21]

Another possible effect of health reform on abortion services is to make more obstetrician/gynecologists available for this work. This may occur because of the emphasis on service by primary care physicians and mid-level practitioners that will inevitably be part of new health plans – again, because of the cost-saving implications of relying on nonspecialists. In short, health reform will undoubtedly intensify the current trend toward having the routine services that in the past were the province of ob/gyns, such as pelvic exams, prenatal visits, and contraceptive services, be delivered by others. Some of these displaced specialists, one might assume, will turn to at least part-time abortion work.[22]

RESPONSES OF THE MEDICAL COMMUNITY
TO THE PROVIDER SHORTAGE

Whatever the eventual resolution of all these issues, the medical community in the United States has a considerable capacity to address the problems of abortion provision and especially the present crisis in the number of providers. A symposium held in 1990, jointly sponsored by the National Abortion Federation and the American College of Obstetricians and Gynecologists, was one of the most significant formal attempts to date to address the provider shortage.[23] This gathering resulted in a number of recommendations intended both to increase the pool of abortion providers and to improve their working conditions.

The inconsistent approach to abortion among residency programs in obstetrics and gynecology was a key concern of the symposium. As mentioned in earlier chapters, abortion training is not routinely required of ob/gyn residents, and nearly half of all graduating ob/gyn residents finish their studies without having performed a first trimester abortion. Participants in the symposium suggested a number of ways to integrate abortion care into the required ob/gyn curriculum (while maintaining an "opt-out" clause for those with religious or moral objections to abortion). The symposium recommended that relevant professional organizations (such as the American Board of Obstetrics and Gynecology) incorporate, as a matter of course, questions about abortion procedures on written and oral examinations, and, most significantly, that the accrediting body for these residencies (the Residency Review Committee for Obstetrics and Gynecology of the Accreditation Council of Graduate Medical Education) should require abortion training at all ob/gyn residency programs. In the several years since the symposium, support has been increasing within ob/gyn circles for such mandated training in abortion, and this requirement was eventually approved by the ACGME in early 1995.[24]

The symposium further noted the problem that, since most abortions now take place in outpatient facilities, the in-hospital rotations of most ob/gyn residents do not provide sufficient experience in abortion. Thus, participants recommended both the creation (in some cases, restoration) of hospital administered outpatient abortion facilities, and the development of formal training relationships between residency programs and freestanding clinics in their communities.

Physicians and physicians-in-training who are not obstetricians-gynecologists constitute another pool of potential abortion providers. Some family practice physicians – Henry Morgentaler, David Bennett, and a number of others interviewed for this study – have long been providing abortions but have had to make their own arrangements, essentially, to receive the necessary training. Some within family practice are now pressing their relevant professional associations to make abortion training available. In response both to the needs of physicians in fields that do not offer abortion training, and to ob/gyn residents whose own programs do not have such a provision, a number of Planned Parenthood centers as well as independent clinics around the country have begun to develop their own training programs, a model that may well spread.

Finally, midlevel practitioners – especially physician assistants, nurse midwives, and nurse practitioners – are yet another pool from which to recruit abortion providers. The NAF-ACOG symposium recommended training midlevels to do earlier abortions, under physician supervision, and the executive board of the College recently endorsed this point.[25] In making this case, advocates point to Vermont, where physician assistants (PAs) associated with the Vermont Women's Health Center have performed abortions since 1972. The Center now provides about half of all abortions taking place in the state, and the PAs at the Center provide training in abortion technique to ob/gyn residents from the University of Vermont. A two-year study of over twenty-five hundred abortions at the Center – half of which were performed by PAs, and half by physicians – found no difference in complication rates between the two groups.[26]

To be sure, the various proposals mentioned above to expand the pool of abortion providers will not be simple to implement. Each of the relevant professional associations has constituencies that will raise objections, for various reasons, to expanding abortion training. Within each of the non-ob/gyn groups – which until now have largely avoided the abortion issue – some will speak against incorporating abortion training because of the moral objections of some members; probably more objections will be raised because of a desire to protect the field in question from the controversy inevitably associated with abortion.

Furthermore, the above proposals are likely to generate a certain amount of conflict *between* different professional groups, a conflict which transcends the abortion issue *per se*. The concept of expanding the pool of abortion providers inevitably runs up against longstanding, often tense debates within medicine about the appropriate division of labor between specialist and nonspecialist and between physician and nonphysician.[27] Family physicians taking on functions that typically have been the province of ob/gyn specialists has been difficult enough for some within medicine; the notion that midlevel practitioners might perform some surgical procedures will likely be seen as heresy by a larger group of physicians, both specialists and nonspecialists. Therefore, though some within obstetrics and gynecology may be only too happy to have others take on the abortion "problem" and release their own field from this burden, others may raise objections that speak more to the protection of professional boundaries than to a commitment to abortion.

There is, moreover, an arguably contradictory element in the simultaneous call for more abortion training within the specialty of obstetrics and gynecology *and* among other physicians and midlevel practitioners. If abortion apparently can be so safely delivered by midlevels and general practice physicians, then what is the logic of incorporating the procedure into an already crowded specialty residency? One response to this contradiction is that ob/gyns and other physicians will always be needed to supervise midlevel practice, attend to complications, and perform later, more technically challenging abortions. Indeed, numerous examples of procedures done by both ob/gyns and nonspecialists already exist. The involvement of midwives in births, for example, has not kept ob/gyns out of obstetrics. Nonetheless, a broadened vision of the pool of potential abortion providers may fuel the tendencies of some within obstetrics and gynecology to pull even further away from a commitment to abortion practice.

It is not clear, at this writing, how successful this call for the recruitment of additional abortion providers from the ranks of midlevel practitioners will be. On the one hand, it is reasonable to anticipate both ideological and bureaucratic resistance to such a change; on the other hand, the larger health reform discussions now under way will inevitably lead to cost-saving pressures for more health services offered by primary care physicians and midlevel practitioners. And the impressive safety record compiled to date by PAs in Vermont and elsewhere makes a very persuasive case for the abilities of nonphysicians to competently perform abortions. Perhaps the best prediction possible at the moment is to visualize a future in which abortion services remain dominated by ob/gyns, but are increasingly offered by providers from other fields as well, with training taking place not only in hospital-based clinics but increasingly in freestanding clinics, and under the aegis of groups such as Planned Parenthood. Assuming that state laws will continue to be interpreted to permit nonphysicians to perform abortions, as several recent key decisions have established,[28] then we can anticipate that interested PAs, nurse-midwives, and nurse practitioners will be able to individually arrange abortion training, even before it is formally offered within their own professional groups.

An expanded pool from which to recruit future abortion providers would mean several things. Most fundamentally, of course, abortion would be more accessible in currently underserved areas. But more providers would also mean that those committed to abortion practice will not have to sacrifice other aspects of medical care that they find gratifying. Two important points that emerged from the interviews for this book are, first, that in spite of their strong ideological commitment to abortion, most providers find the procedure itself to be technically unchallenging, often tedious; and second, that most of those whose careers revolve exclusively, or nearly exclusively, around abortion express considerable wistfulness for opportunities forgone – for example, the practice of obstetrics or family medicine. To express these findings another way, those with the most positive responses to abortion work tend to be those who combine it with a range of other medical activities.

To address the shortage, therefore, it is not enough just to increase the number of recruits to the field. In order to sustain the commitment of those who undertake abortion provision, the working conditions that characterize this field must be changed as well. Certainly until the arrival of RU-486, and perhaps even afterwards, most abortions in the foreseeable future will continue to take place in freestanding clinics. Thus these clinics will face the greatest burden to accommodate creatively the needs of would-be providers.

If many full-time providers find abortion work technically unchallenging and are regretful that they are not involved in other aspects of medicine, then obviously clinics must be prepared to hire a number of physicians who wish to work only part time, rather than the arguably more convenient full-time providers (a policy already under way in many clinics). Beyond this, those interviewed for this study have suggested some other directions for change in clinic operations. Recall, for example, Ethan Stevenson's rueful comment, in the last chapter, that his work in a freestanding clinic made him feel like "a fool at the end of the curette." Stevenson was referring to a problem echoed by others in this study – that as counseling in the clinic movement developed into a specialized function to be performed by specially trained staff, many physicians increasingly came to miss a sense of relationship with the abortion patient and to feel themselves to be merely "hired technicians." For many, though certainly not all, providers, it is dissatisfying to have their interaction with a patient typically limited to the ten minutes or so required for the abortion itself. To deal with this problem, clinics must take doctors' preferences into account and allow those who wish to to take part in counseling as well.

Increasing the repertoire of clinic medical procedures as well as enhancing research opportunities are other possible incentives that clinics might offer to attract physicians. The NAF-ACOG symposium, for example, suggested that adding procedures such as colposcopies and other outpatient surgeries would serve as inducement for some to affiliate with such clinics.[29] Freestanding clinics vary widely in their support of practitioners' research and publishing interests. Again, we can recall Ethan Stevenson's disappointment when he was dissuaded from pursuing a research program while employed at such a clinic. Stevenson's disappointment stands in sharp contrast to the immense gratification reported by Jane Hodgson, in chapter 1, with the research opportunities available in the clinic she served as medical director in Washington, D.C. Certainly not all potential abortion providers are interested in doing medical research (nor are all clinics large enough to support such ventures), but if more clinics aggressively pursued university affiliation, and made clear their readiness to cooperate with research ventures, there is reason to believe that more physicians would find these clinics attractive places to work.

Finally, in order to address the provider shortage, clinics must confront the complex question of adequate payment. As has been clear throughout this book, the relationship between abortion and money is uniquely charged. The physicians interviewed for this book became involved in abortion at a time when illegal abortions were closely associated in the public mind with the greed and exploitation of "back alley butchers." We have seen the various ways in which these physicians showed their awareness of the tainted association of abortion and money. Some who provided abortions before *Roe*, such as Simon Ross, decided not to take any payment whatsoever, feeling that such a policy would put them on safer legal ground if they were apprehended. Others, such as Henry Morgentaler, who similarly anticipated that he would be accused of profiteering, made every effort to set fees as reasonably as possible and established sliding-scale fees for poor women. To be sure, these cautious policies were not adopted simply to protect themselves, if necessary, against accusations of greed. A prime motivation was their compassion for desperate women and a corresponding rage at the unethical abortionists who exploited this desperation. Virtually everyone in this study who performed illegal abortions routinely provided free abortions for indigent women. But the point remains that these "conscience" physicians felt obliged to protect themselves against the suspicion of greed.

Like other aspects of the history of abortion provision, the presumed venality of abortionists in the pre-*Roe* era continues to inform the present in subtle, and sometimes not so subtle, ways. A major rhetorical device of the contemporary antiabortion movement is to denounce the profit motives allegedly driving the abortion "industry." While the public may periodically decry doctors' high salaries in general, there seems to be a special valence attached to money made from performing abortions. Even two decades after *Roe*, many providers seem defensive about monetary compensation from this work. Periodically, in the course of conducting the interviews for this book, I would be told by a participant, "You know, I'm not in this work for the money," even though I had not raised the issue. I doubt that had I been interviewing a group of cardiovascular surgeons, whose average annual income is in fact far higher than that of the ob/gyns and family practitioners in this study, I would have heard such spontaneous disclaimers about compensation.[30]

In reality, in marked contrast to most other medical procedures, the cost of an abortion (and the fees paid to a physician) has actually fallen over time. David Grimes, a leading student of abortion services, has pointed out that the average cost of a first trimester abortion in 1991 – below $300 – was, in 1991 dollars, about half the cost of the procedure at the time of legalization. While doctors working in clinics in 1973 were typically paid about $50 per case (about $190 in today's dollars), they currently receive only $30 to $50 in today's dollars for each operation.[31]

This current low rate of remuneration to abortion providers in freestanding clinics has several sources. One, as suggested, is a continuing need to distance contemporary abortion provision from an unsavory history of financial exploitation. But current abortion costs also reflect the quite unique history of patient advocacy among the first cohort of legal abortion providers – a history one would be hard pressed to find in other medical services. As we have seen earlier in this book, when the Clergy Consultation Service began working with physicians in the immediate pre-*Roe* era, one of their primary goals was to make abortions as affordable as possible. When the first freestanding clinics opened in New York and Washington, D.C. in the early 1970s, again a primary goal was to deliver the best possible care at the lowest possible price. In particular, the promoters of the clinic model contrasted the cost of an outpatient abortion to that of one requiring several days of hospitalization and general anesthesia. In New York, especially, as numerous clinics opened to meet the huge demands of a then national market, several feminist health organizations established their own referral services, with the cost of an abortion being one prime criterion for approval.

Increasing abortion providers' compensation would obviously mean raising the cost of an abortion, a step that many clinic administrators would find difficult, especially given the present political impossibility in most states of obtaining subsidized abortions for the poor. (Currently, only fifteen states continue to provide Medicaid-funded abortions.) Furthermore, given the current atmosphere of health reform, when there are tremendous pressures on the medical system as a whole to contain costs, this is not a propitious moment to suggest raising fees in any area of health care. Yet the typically low rates of remuneration for abortion provision in freestanding clinics undoubtedly discourage some from entering this field, and clinics may well be increasingly pressured to raise fees in order to be able to pay providers more. As Grimes has written of the provider shortage, "Paying clinicians appropriately for their services will likely overcome much of the current reluctance. . . . Inequitable compensation for this service denigrates its value to the patient and to society."[32]

AFFIRMING ABORTION PRACTICE

All the strategies described above–pressuring ob/gyn residencies to provide abortion training, targeting midlevel practitioners for this work, improving the pay and working conditions for providers in clinics–hold promise for addressing the shortage of abortion providers in the United States. But the most fundamental change needed within the medical community to deal with this problem is one that cannot be simply addressed at the "policy" level. Rather, I speak of a full-fledged attitudinal change. The crisis of abortion provision will not be solved until the medical community as a whole confronts its historic ambivalence about abortion providers. That majority of U.S. physicians who consider themselves "pro-choice" must acknowledge the inadequacy of supporting "abortion" while allowing the abortion provider to remain marginalized–and often victimized–within medical circles. This pro-choice majority should affirm at every opportunity the full membership of their abortion-providing colleagues in the wider medical community. A failure to do this will not only lead to the avoidance of abortion work by qualified providers, but, just as worrisome, will make it more likely that some of the worst contemporary medical practitioners will come to fill this void in abortion services.

The notorious case of Abu Hayat, a physician who practiced in the New York area, illustrates this point well. Hayat practiced in a low-income neighborhood serving largely immigrant women and was accused in 1989 of both egregious medical and ethical practices. Among the various charges he faced were performing an illegal abortion of a 30- to 32-week fetus, which ultimately resulted in the patient giving birth to an infant whose arm had been severed; perforating a teenaged patient's uterus, which led to infection and the patient's death; and stopping an abortion in mid-procedure when the patient's husband was unable to come up with the additional cash the doctor demanded.[33] While antiabortion forces predictably use the Hayat case to declaim against all who provide abortion, the pro-choice analysis is that such cases are the tragic and inevitable result both of abortion provision having become so separate from mainstream medicine, and of the inaccessibility of reputable abortion services for poor women.

To date, thankfully, there have been very few cases similar to Abu Hayat's, but, as in the pre-*Roe* era, the inadequate number of abortion providers leaves the field open to the inept and exploitative. This makes it all the more imperative for the medical community to actively support that vast majority of providers who are medically competent and ethically sound. Such support means helping providers in their numerous struggles, not only against protestors in the streets, but against opponents within medicine. Physicians as a group may not have the power, by themselves, to stop antiabortion terrorism at the clinic; they *do* have the power, however, to end much of the unjustified harassment that many abortion providers suffer within the medical profession. When some hospital boards attempt to disaffiliate with physicians because they perform abortions, when some state medical boards appear to pursue their oversight functions more zealously with abortion providers than with others, when hospitals refuse to offer back-up services to local clinics, when abortion providing physicians are denied promotion in academic medicine, when editorial boards and program committees of professional associations appear to be biased against abortion-related material – in these and in many other instances, pro-choice physicians must take a stand and ascertain that such treatment is not driven by ideological opposition to abortion.

Physicians who are morally opposed to abortion can be urged by

their peers to adopt an attitude of greater tolerance toward their colleagues who perform a procedure that is legal and whose public
health benefits have been amply documented. Rather than opposing
these providers by trying to sabotage their abortion activity – and
sometimes, their careers as a whole, as occurred to some of those interviewed for this study – antiabortion physicians would arguably do
better to seek common ground with their abortion providing colleagues in attempting to prevent unintended pregnancies. Again and
again in this study, participants expressed frustration with a health
care system in which contraceptive research was such a low priority,
and with a society in which contraceptive practices were so inadequate. For many abortion providers, one of the saddest aspects of
the abortion conflict within medicine is precisely the distraction it
causes from the more fundamental task of addressing the "insanity,"
to repeat Daniel Fieldstone's words, of over half of all pregnancies in
the United States being reported as unintended.

A NEW GENERATION OF ABORTION PROVIDERS

But even should contraceptive practices improve, some abortions
will always be necessary. And thus, we must return to the questions
that were posed at the beginning of the chapter: Who will provide
abortions in the future, now that the providers who came of age in the
pre-*Roe* era enter retirement? What will secure the commitment of a
new generation of health professionals, doctors who have never attended women dying of illegal abortions?

Part of the answer lies in widespread education about older physicians' experiences, and several groups are involved in efforts to sys-
tematically inform contemporary medical students about pre-*Roe*
history. While such activities are very important, they are unlikely,
by themselves, to motivate large numbers of young physicians to become involved in abortion provision. Each generation of activists –
and physicians willing to engage with such a divisive social issue as
abortion are indisputably "activists" – experiences its own defining
moments. And just as the death of women in emergency rooms was
such a defining experience for older abortion providers, there are indications that the murders of abortion providers and other recent ex-

tremist antiabortion activity are playing the same role today for many contemporary medical students.

Since David Gunn's death in March 1993, there has been a significant mobilization among pro-choice medical students across the country. "Medical Students for Choice," a new national organization, has contacts in over one hundred medical schools. One of its first activities was to circulate a petition (which ultimately gathered over three thousand signatures) among medical students all over the country, demanding that abortion training be a required component in ob/gyn residency programs. On individual campuses, students similarly press for inclusion of abortion information in the curricula, and for abortion to be offered through their university's health services. In response to the notorious "Bottom Feeders" pamphlet, a compilation of vulgar jokes directed at abortion providers, which was recently mailed to medical students in the United States by an antiabortion group, medical students at the University of California at San Francisco raised funds that were donated to the National Abortion Federation. In a letter to the publishers of this pamphlet, the UCSF students wrote, "If your intentions included intimidating future abortion providers . . . then you failed. In fact, 'Bottom Feeders' has sparked effective discussions on campus about how to insure access to safe, legal abortion for every woman who wants one."[34]

The "conscience" physicians who became involved in abortion before *Roe* and the activists among the current generation of medical students and residents came of age in quite different legal and political environments. The former literally had to break the law to provide abortion; the latter prepare to provide abortion in an atmosphere in which, although abortion is legal, it has been politicized and made dangerous in a way not dreamed of in the pre-*Roe* era. But the continuity between these two groups is their strong sense of commitment to their patients. As the older physicians once refused to jeopardize the health of their patients in the face of unjust laws, so now a new generation dedicated to women's health care refuses to be deterred by the actions of terrorists. And given the evidence suggesting a higher degree of support for abortion services among female physicians,[35] the steadily increasing number of women in medical schools in the 1980s and 1990s very likely means a larger pool of those who plan to pursue abortion training.

Thus, in spite of the serious situation of abortion services in the contemporary United States that has been documented throughout this book, we can end on a note of cautious optimism. Recently approved changes in the standards for ob/gyn residency programs, which mandate training in abortion techniques, mean that more specialists than before will be familiar with the procedure. The near-certainty of the eventual distribution in the United States of RU-486 and other forms of medical abortion will mean abortion services will be dispersed throughout the health care system, a development that will be especially significant for women living in areas where there are no providers of surgical abortion. Furthermore, the organizational and legal steps now under way to open up abortion work to midlevel practitioners may, ultimately, considerably increase the number of abortion providers. But even with an infusion of new providers from the ranks of midlevels, abortion for the foreseeable future will remain under the supervision and control of physicians. Thus, the most promising sign of all for those who wish to see abortion remain available is that a new generation of medical students – mobilized not only by antiabortion extremism but also by the ideas of gender equality that have permeated U.S. campuses for the last twenty years – appears ready to continue the work of an earlier generation. It is the responsibility of the medical profession to assure that these young physicians will not have to pay the price of professional isolation for acting on their consciences.

Afterword

In the spring of 1994, during the annual meeting of the National Abortion Federation in Cincinnati, a group of about twenty-five, mostly female, medical students gather for an informal encounter with seven abortion-providing physicians, all women in their thirties and forties. The students speak about both their pull toward eventual abortion provision, as well as their hesitations. They raise fears about personal safety, and, in some cases, the disapproval of family members. Some also worry about the career consequences of being identified with abortion provision. On the other hand, all believe fervently in safe and accessible abortion as a necessary component of women's health care. One student volunteers that were it not for the availability of abortion when she was a high school student, she would not have achieved her lifelong dream of medical school. All are outraged by the attempts of "fanatics" to interfere with medical services. What the young students seem to most want from the older women in the room is to grasp how the latter "pull it all together" – that is, in the face of such intense social conflict about abortion, how do these providers attend to their personal safety, deal with their families' concerns, sustain a satisfying medical practice, lead a "normal" life?

One by one, the physicians in the room respond to the students. First, they describe their work situations. Several of them work full time in clinics, providing both abortions and gynecological services. Others combine abortion provision with either family practice or obstetrics. All acknowledge the seriousness with which they take threats to their safety. One doctor confides that she wears a bullet-proof vest while driving to and from work. Another jokes about such vests "not doing much for her figure" but then, more seriously, explains why she considered that option for herself and then rejected it. The group also engages in some joking discussion – *albeit* with a serious undertone – about which breed of dog is the most fearsome, and hence the most effective for home security. There is a quite poignant discussion about the steps they take to reassure family members, especially young children. Most, however, report tremendous support from their families; the one exception is a Midwest physician who speaks of past conflict with her former "fundamentalist in-laws."

Predictably, each of the physicians voices strong ideological support for abortion. One expresses her view that "motherhood should be a sacrament, not a punishment for one sexual encounter." Another woman, drawing on her ten years of experience as a family practitioner, speaks of her conviction that being an unwanted child is a huge risk factor for serious health problems later in life. She goes on to say that it is "unnacceptable" medical practice to force a woman to have a baby she doesn't want. Several refer not only to their own abortions, but also to other reproductive events in their lives, such as childbirth and adoption, as occasions which viscerally reinforced for them the importance of making a full range of reproductive choices available to all women.

Somewhat less predictably, however, given the turbulence and occasional violence surrounding abortion services, each of the physicians present speaks eloquently of how ultimately gratifying it is, nevertheless, to be involved in this aspect of health care. One provider states, "There is nothing else I do in my medical practice where people look me in the eye, in quite the same way, and say 'thank you.' I feel I am empowering women." Another, nodding agreement with this statement, says to the students, "You will be hard pressed to find similar passion among doctors in other fields. We are so lucky to have found work we love." A third continues the discussion, also addressing the students: "You ask how I can do this work? For me, the question is, how could I not?"

Notes

PREFACE

1. The figure of 1.2 million illegal abortions was first cited at a landmark 1955 conference on abortion (to be discussed further in chapter 2), when a committee chaired by the biostatistician Christopher Tietze concluded: "a plausible estimate of the frequency of induced abortion in the United States could be as low as 200,000 and as high as 1.2 million per year." In Mary Calderone, ed., *Abortion in the United States: Report of a Conference Sponsored by the Planned Parenthood Federation* (New York: Hoeber-Harper, 1958), p. 180. This figure retained credibility in most medical and social science circles in the years leading up to *Roe* and was restated by several speakers at another major abortion conference held in 1968 (also to be discussed in chapter 2). Also in 1968, Michael Burnhill, a physician/demographer, estimated the number of illegal abortions in the United States to be between 650,000 and 1.3 million annually. In Robert Hall, ed., *Abortion in a Changing World*, vol. 2 (New York: Columbia University Press, 1970), p. 44.

For an estimate that physicians provided one third of all illegal abortions, see Daniel Callahan, ed., *Abortion: Law, Choice, Morality* (New York: Macmillan, 1970), p. 131.

2. Rickie Solinger, *The Abortionist: A Woman Against the Law* (New York: Free Press, 1994). The focus of Solinger's book is Ruth Barnett, a Portland-based lay abortionist, who, in some fifty years of abortion provision, performed an estimated forty thousand abortions with no deaths and, apparently, relatively few injuries.

3. Warren Hern, Letter to the Editor, *New York Times*, September 7, 1993, p. A22.

INTRODUCTION

1. *Planned Parenthood of Southeastern Pennsylvania v. Casey*, 112 SCt 2791. The implications of this case for contemporary abortion provision are discussed in chapter 7.

2. Stanley Henshaw and Jennifer Van Vort, "Abortion Services in the United States, 1991 and 1992," *Family Planning Perspectives* 26 (1994): 100–106, 112; *Abortion Factbook, 1992* (New York: Alan Guttmacher Institute, 1992), pp. 56–57.

3. The most recent (1991) figures on routine abortion training – 12 percent for first trimester procedures and 6 percent for second trimester ones – show a decline from 22 percent in each case in 1985, when such a survey of ob/gyn residency programs previously took place. Trent McKay, "Abortion Training in U.S. Obstetrics and Gynecology Residency Programs: A Follow-Up Study," *Family Planning Perspectives* (in press); Philip Darney, Uta Landy, S. MacPherson, and R. Sweet, "Abortion Training in U.S. Obstetrics and Gynecology Programs," *Family Planning Perspectives* 19 (1987): 158–62. The Columbia University study is reported in Carolyn Westhoff, Frances Marks, and Allan Rosenfeld, "Residency Training in Contraception, Sterilization, and Abortion," *Obstetrics and Gynecology* 81 (1993): 311–14.

Henshaw and Van Vort report in "Abortion Services in the United States, 1991–92" that 1,529,000 abortions were performed in 1992, the lowest number since 1979. These 1992 figures represent an abortion rate of 26 per 1,000 women of reproductive age, in contrast to a high of 29 per 1,000 women in 1981. The authors offer no one overriding reason for this decline. Besides the increasing inaccessibility of abortion services for many women, especially those in nonmetropolitan areas, the authors also suggest other possible contributing factors such as the increasing acceptability of out-of-wedlock births, a higher rate of contraceptive usage, and changing attitudes toward abortion (pp. 106, 112). This drop in abortions garnered front-page, headline coverage in the *New York Times*. Tamar Lewin, "Abortions in U.S. Hit 13-Year Low, A Study Reports," *New York Times*, June 16, 1994, pp. A1, A11.

4. "Deaths from legal abortion declined fivefold between 1973 and 1985 (from 3.3 deaths to 0.4 death per 100,000 procedures), reflecting increased physician education and skills, improvements in medical technology, and, notably, the earlier termination of pregnancy. . . . Legal-abortion mortality between 1979 and 1985 was 0.6 death per 100,000 procedures, more than 10 times lower than the 9.1 maternal deaths per 100,000 live births between 1979 and 1986." Council on Scientific Affairs, American Medical Association, "In-

duced Termination of Pregnancy Before and After *Roe v. Wade*:," *Journal of the American Medical Association* 268 (1992): 3231–39.

5. Neil Nevitte, William Brandon, and Lori Davis found, in their examination of Gallup polls, that in June 1992, 13 percent of respondents felt abortion should be "illegal in all circumstances," 48 percent felt it should be "legal under certain circumstances," and 34 percent felt abortion should be "legal under any circumstance." "The American Abortion Controversy: Lessons from Cross-national Evidence," *Politics and the Life Sciences* 12 (1993): 21. As an example of abortion polls giving quite different results when questions are phrased differently, the Harris and Gallup polls, taken shortly before the *Webster* case in 1989, found that 57 to 58 percent were opposed to the overturning of *Roe v. Wade*; however, in another poll during the same period, when the question was phrased as agreement or disagreement with the following statement, "Abortion is a private issue between a woman, her family and her doctor [and] the government should not be involved," 73 percent of respondents agreed. "Majority of Americans Oppose Overturning *Roe v. Wade* and Banning Abortions Outright, Polls Show," *Family Planning Perspectives* 21 (1989): 114–15. *Webster v. Reproductive Health Services*, U.S. 490 (1989).

On ob/gyns, see American College of Obstetricians and Gynecologists, "Abortion Attitudes: Little Change in 14 Years," Washington, D.C., August 1985, and "ACOG Poll: Ob-Gyns' Support for Abortion Unchanged Since 1971," *Family Planning Perspectives* 17 (1985): 275.

6. Henshaw and Van Vort, *Abortion Factbook*, p. 48; National Abortion Federation, Washington, D.C., "Incidents of Violence and Disruption Against Providers, 1992, 1993." On the Brookline deaths, see John Kifner, "Gunman Kills 2 at Abortion Clinics in Boston Suburb," *New York Times*, December 31, 1994, pp. A1, A8. The murders of Gunn, Britton, and Barrett will be further discussed in chapter 7.

7. Drawing on data collected by the National Abortion Federation, Dallas Blanchard points out that in 1984, there were thirty reported instances of bombing and arson at abortion clinics, in contrast to only a handful in each of the preceding years since 1977. Blanchard attributes this upsurge in 1984 to the mounting frustration among antiabortionists with the Reagan administration, which, rhetoric notwithstanding, had done little to ban abortion. Dallas Blanchard, *The Anti-Abortion Movement and the Rise of the Religious Right* (New York: Twayne, 1994), pp. 53–58.

8. Jacqueline Forrest, of the Alan Guttmacher Institute, estimated in the mid-1980s that some 46 percent of American women will have had an abor-

tion by the age of forty-five. "Unintended Pregnancy Among American Women," *Family Planning Perspectives* 19 (1987): 76–77.

9. My approach to the study of work and occupations has been most deeply influenced by the writings of the late Everett Hughes. His essays on this subject have been collected in *The Sociological Eye*, vols. 1 and 2 (Chicago: Aldine, 1971).

1. "I'VE BEEN LUCKY TO HAVE BEEN PART OF THIS"

1. For an account of Hodgson's trial, including its relationship to other key abortion cases in the courts at that period, see David Garrow, *Liberty and Sexuality: The Right to Privacy and the Making of Roe v. Wade* (New York: Macmillan, 1994), pp. 428–30, 466–68, 471, 474, 476, 479.

2. Jane E. Hodgson, "The Office Use of the Frog Test for Pregnancy," *Journal of the American Medical Association* 154 (1953): 271–74.

3. As I will discuss in greater detail in chapter 2, therapeutic abortion committees, widely in use in U.S. hospitals from the late 1940s through the *Roe* decision, were organizational mechanisms established to monitor the requests for hospital abortions.

4. For a recent account of such maternity homes, see Rickie Solinger, *Wake Up Little Susie: Single Pregnancy and Race before Roe v. Wade* (New York: Routledge, 1992).

5. Jane E. Hodgson, "Therapeutic Abortions in Medical Perspective," *Minnesota Medicine* 53 (1970): 757.

6. Jane E. Hodgson, "Teenage Mothers," *Minnesota Medicine* 55 (1972): 49.

7. Lucas's role in several key abortion rights cases of the 1960s and 1970s, including *Roe v. Wade*, is discussed extensively in Garrow, *Liberty and Privacy*. Lucas initially drew the attention of many in the abortion rights movement, including Hodgson, when he published a landmark law review article which suggested that "privacy" arguments could be applied to abortion, drawing on the 1965 Supreme Court case, *Griswold v. Connecticut*, 381 U.S. 479, which similarly used privacy arguments to establish the rights of married persons to use birth control. Roy Lucas, "Constitutional Limitations on the Enforcement and Administration of State Abortion Statutes," *North Carolina Law Review* 46 (1968): 730–78.

8. Tietze and his wife, Sarah Lewit, conducted one of the first large-scale studies measuring the safety of outpatient abortion. Christopher Tietze and

Sarah Lewit, "Joint Program for the Study of Abortion," *Studies in Family Planning* 3 (1972): 97–124.

9. Jane E. Hodgson, "Abortion: The Law and Reality in 1970," *The Mayo Alumnus* (1970): 1–4.

10. Jane E. Hodgson, "Major Complications of 20,248 Consecutive First Trimester Abortions: Problems of Fragmented Care," *Advances in Planned Parenthood* 9 (1975): 52–59.

11. Jane E. Hodgson, "Response to Dr. Fehr's Article on Abortion Complications," *Minnesota Medicine* 56 (1973): 698–99.

12. *Harris v. McCrae*, 448 U.S. 297 (1980); *Hodgson v. Minnesota*, 497 U.S. 417 (1990).

13. Jane Hodgson, "The Role of the Freestanding Clinic in Providing Community Abortion Services," *Proceedings of the Annual Meeting of the Canadian Public Health Association* (Ottawa: Canadian Public Health Association, 1974), pp. 328–36. The case of Henry Morgentaler is discussed in chapter 4.

14. Jane E. Hodgson and Renee Ward, "Provision and Organization of Abortion and Sterilization Services in the United States," in J. Hodgson, ed., *Abortion and Sterilization: Medical and Social Aspects* (New York: Grune and Stratton, 1981), p. 538.

15. For an account of Hodgson's commute to perform abortions in Duluth, see Cynthia Gorney, "Hodgson's Choice: A Long, Cold Abortion Fight," Washington *Post*, November 29, 1989, pp. B1, B6–9.

2. U.S. MEDICINE AND THE
MARGINALIZATION OF ABORTION

1. This following discussion of the history of abortion, and particularly the role of physicians in the antiabortion campaign of the nineteenth century, draws on Kristin Luker, *Abortion and the Politics of Motherhood* (Berkeley: University of California Press, 1984); James Mohr, *Abortion in America: The Origins and Evolution of National Policy, 1800–1900* (New York: Oxford University Press, 1978); Rosalind P. Petchesky, *Abortion and Women's Choice*, rev. ed. (Boston: Northeastern University Press, 1990); and Carroll Smith-Rosenberg, "The Abortion Movement and the AMA, 1850–1880," in her *Disorderly Conduct: Visions of Gender in Victorian America* (New York: Knopf, 1985), pp. 217–44.

2. As Smith-Rosenberg writes, in "The Abortion Movement and the

AMA," "Abortion-related ads provided a lucrative source of income for the new urban newspapers. By the 1840s and 1850s, ads for abortafacients filled their pages. . . . Physicians, midwives, and many others who specialized in gynecological ailments, whatever their formal training, set up special clinics, advertised their fee scales, solicited customers, printed cards, even sent business agents out into agrarian areas and smaller towns to solicit business. . . . By mid-century, abortion had become a big business" (pp. 225–26).

3. Two of the strongest statements within contemporary feminist scholarship of this connection between reproductive conflicts and gender politics are Petchesky, *Abortion and Woman's Choice*, and Linda Gordon, *Woman's Body, Woman's Right* (Baltimore: Penguin, 1977). As Petchesky writes with respect to the abortion conflict in our own time, *"abortion is the fulcrum of a much broader ideological struggle in which the very meanings of the family, the state, motherhood, and young women's sexuality are contested"* (p. xi, emphasis hers).

4. Quoted in Smith-Rosenberg, "The Abortion Movement and the AMA," pp. 236–37. For a contemporary antiabortion statement, which presents the abortion-seeking woman in a similar light, see Connaught Marshner, *The New Traditional Woman* (Washington, D.C.: Free Congress Research and Educational Foundation, 1982).

5. Mohr, *Abortion in America*, p. 254.

6. As with estimates of the frequency of illegal abortion, estimates of death from illegal abortion have been highly contested, with the antiabortion movement, in particular, accusing the pro-choice movement of inflating the figures. Numerous commentators have pointed out how difficult it is to make such an estimate, given the likelihood that many abortion deaths were listed as something else, in order to mask the shame associated with illegal abortion. Writing in 1948, Christopher Tietze suggested a figure of approximately one thousand abortion deaths per year, while a well-regarded study in 1962 offered the estimate of five thousand deaths per year. Christopher Tietze, "Abortion as a Cause of Death," *Journal of Public Health* 38 (1948): 1434–41; Zad Leavy and Jerome M. Kummer, "Criminal Abortion: Human Hardship and Unyielding Laws," *Southern California Law Review* 35 (1962): 126.

7. National Abortion Rights Action League, *Facing a Future Without Choice: A Report on Reproductive Liberty in America* (Washington, D.C.: National Abortion Rights Action League, 1992), p. 16.

8. Ellen Messer and Kathryn May, *Back Rooms: Voices from the Illegal Abortion Era* (New York: St. Martin's Press), pp. 148–49.

9. National Abortion Rights Action League, *Facing a Future without*

Choice, p. 15. See also Jerome Bates and Edward Zawadzki, *Criminal Abortion: A Study in Medical Sociology* (Springfield, Ill.: Charles C. Thomas, 1964). Yet the founders of the Clergy Consultation Service on Abortion – whose organization, as will be discussed in subsequent chapters, ultimately arranged 100,000 abortion referrals – disagreed with the view that illegal abortion was dominated by organized crime. "One of the interesting phenomena of the illicit abortion business in the United States was that the 'Mafia' or the underworld syndicate never moved into the field and dominated it, even though it was a multimillion-dollar business annually. . . . The only place that seemed an exception to this rule was the state of New Jersey, where there was evidence of outside controls over doctors and 'middlemen.'" Arlene Carmen and Howard Moody, *Abortion Counseling and Social Change: The Story of the Clergy Consultation Service on Abortion* (Valley Forge, Pa.: Judson, 1973), pp. 16–17.

10. On the relation of the criminal justice system to illegal abortion, see Bates and Zawadzki, *Criminal Abortion*; B. James George, "Current Abortion Laws: Proposals and Movements for Reform," in David Smith, ed., *Abortion and the Law* (Cleveland: Case Western Reserve Press, 1967), pp. 1–36, and "The Evolving Law of Abortion," *Western Reserve Law Review* 23 (1972): 708–55; Betty Sarvis and Hyman Rodman, *The Abortion Controversy* (New York: Columbia University Press, 1974), pp. 29–40. As Sarvis and Rodman note, "Although the loss of license for performing criminal abortions is a relatively rare occurrence, the fear inspired up until 1973 by labeling the practice of unlawful abortion as unprofessional conduct should not be underestimated. [A study] reported that of 208 medical licenses revoked in 1967 in thirty-one states, twenty-three related to professional competence which included only abortion and narcotics violation" (p. 35).

Rickie Solinger, in explaining the higher prosecution rate of lay women abortionists than of male doctors, wrote, "District attorneys often determined that abortion prosecutions were fairly likely to be successful since women abortionists were presumed to be untrained, unskilled, and unprotected. Doctors, on the other hand, were presumed to have skills and resources, and could be assumed to have respectable colleagues who would stand up in court and claim that a given abortion was not criminal, but medically necessary. Such testimony would, of course, undermine a conviction." "Extreme Danger: Woman Abortionists and their Clients Before *Roe v. Wade*," in Joanne Meyerowitz, ed., *Not June Cleaver: Women in the Postwar U.S.* (Philadelphia: Temple University Press, 1994), pp. 335–57.

11. Solinger, in *The Abortionist*, pp. 149–68, traces a police "crackdown" on illegal abortion providers (both physician and lay) in Portland in 1948 – where illegal abortionists had previously operated openly and without

interference – to rising social anxieties about "vice" in the postwar period and, more specifically, to the mayoral campaign in the city that year.

12. Calderone, ed., *Abortion in the United States*, p. 41. For a vivid account of an abortion patient being interrogated by police literally up to the moment of her death, see Leslie Reagan, " 'About to Meet Her Maker': Women, Doctors, Dying Declarations, and the State's Investigation of Abortion, Chicago, 1867–1940," *Journal of American History* 77 (1991): 1240–64.

13. On the Finkbine case, see Luker, *Abortion and the Politics of Motherhood*, pp. 62–65, 78–79, 80, 82, 85, 89; and Finkbine's own account in Alan Guttmacher, ed., *The Case for Legalized Abortion* (Berkeley: Diablo Press, 1967), pp. 15–25.

14. For an account of the San Francisco Nine case, see Lawrence Lader, *Abortion II: Making the Revolution* (Boston: Beacon Press, 1973), pp. 67–69; and Keith Monroe, "How California's Abortion Law Isn't Working," *The New York Times Magazine*, December 29, 1968, pp. 10–11, 17–20. As the *New York Times*' coverage of the incident put it, in a story about a defense fund being organized for the charged physicians, "The prestige and professional connections of the defenders of the doctors is typified in this statement from Dr. Edmund V. Overstreet, vice-chairman of obstetrics at the University of California. 'We do not believe that violation of an archaic statute is unprofessional conduct, nor that it is unprofessional for a physician to conduct himself in accord with the ethics of the community, the wishes of patients and the best medical judgment of doctors.' " Wallace Turner, "Doctors Backed in Abortion Clash," *New York Times*, March 12, 1967, p. A12.

On the number of rubella-caused defects, see Lawrence Tribe, *Abortion: The Clash of Absolutes* (New York: Norton, 1990), p. 37.

15. On the Comstock laws, see James Reed, *The Birth Control Movement and American Society: From Private Vice to Public Virtue* (Princeton: Princeton University Press, 1983), pp. 12, 37–39, 97, 107, 168, 391; and Mohr, *Abortion in America*, pp. 196–99. *Griswold v. Connecticut*, 381 U.S. 479 (1965) and *Eisenstadt v. Baird*, 405 U.S. 438 (1972).

16. On Sanger's life and career generally, and especially on her difficult relationship with the medical profession, see Ellen Chesler, *Woman of Valor: Margaret Sanger and the Birth Control Movement in America* (New York: Simon and Schuster, 1992). On the AMA and birth control, see *ibid.*, p. 374.

'17. *Ibid.*, p. 280. Chesler also cites evidence, pp. 300–303, that staff at Sanger's clinic occasionally made abortion referrals as well (both for "therapeutic abortions" in hospitals and to illegal abortionists) in spite of Sanger's careful public strategy of dissociating birth control from the even more stigmatized subject of abortion.

18. *Ibid.*, p. 279. Reed offers a similar account of professional punishment for involvement with birth control in his discussion of the career of Robert Dickinson, a prominent gynecologist in the first half of the twentieth century and ultimately one of the leading physician advocates of birth control. However, in 1916, early in his career, he refused Sanger's invitation to become publicly identified with her cause, being unwilling, as Reed put it in *The Birth Control Movement and American Society*, to "commit professional suicide by associating with the feminists and radicals who were attacking Comstockery" (p. 46).

19. On this "demographic transition" toward smaller families, see, for example, Peter Lindert, *Fertility and Scarcity in America* (Princeton, N.J.: Princeton University Press, 1978); and Arland Thornton and Deborah Freedman, "The Changing American Family," *Population Bulletin* 38 (1983): 1–43. By these accounts, the larger families of the post–World War II "baby boom" were an anomaly in an otherwise steady pattern of lowered fertility.

20. Luker, *Abortion and the Politics of Motherhood*, pp. 55–56.

21. Alan Guttmacher, "The Genesis of Liberalized Abortion in New York: A Personal Insight," with an update by Irwin Kaiser, in *Abortion, Medicine and the Law*, ed. J. Douglas Butler and David Walbert, 4th ed. (New York: Facts on File, 1992), pp. 546–65. See also the remarks of Guttmacher and other physicians (some of whom were quite critical of the committee system) reported in Robert Hall, ed., *Abortion in a Changing World*, vol. 2, pp. 71–88.

22. Lawrence Lader, *Abortion* (Boston: Beacon Press, 1966), p. 24. On the link between committee-approved abortions and sterilization requirements, and for a severe critique of the workings of the committees as a whole, see Rickie Solinger, " 'A Complete Disaster': Abortion and the Politics of Hospital Abortion Committees, 1950–1970," *Feminist Studies* 19 (1993): 241–68, esp. pp. 257–61.

In a well-known study in the late 1950s, two Stanford law professors submitted a number of hypothetical cases of women seeking abortions to the obstetrical staffs of twenty-six hospitals in Los Angeles and the Bay Area, and found a markedly inconsistent pattern in the responses – giving further weight to the argument that the therapeutic abortion committees were operating arbitrarily. Herbert Packer and Ralph Gampell, "Therapeutic Abortion: A Problem in Law and Medicine," *Stanford Law Review* 11 (1959): 417–55.

23. Garrow, *Liberty and Privacy*, pp. 296–300.

24. Tribe, *Abortion: The Clash of Absolutes*, pp. 36, 42, 50, 71.

25. On the abortion rights movement of the 1960s and 1970s (and particularly the splits between more moderate "reformers" and those advocating repeal), see Lawrence Lader, *Abortion II: Making the Revolution*, and Garrow, *Liberty and Privacy*, chaps. 5 and 6, pp. 270–88. Patricia Maginnis and Laura Phelan were two of the earliest and most visible activists on behalf of abortion rights on the West Coast; among numerous other activities, they published a handbook in 1969 which gave instructions in "do-it-yourself abortions," as well as strategies for gaining a hospital-approved abortion, such as simulating psychoses and simulating hemorrhages. Portions of this handbook have been reprinted in a volume published by the National Woman's Health Network, *Abortion Then and Now: Creative Responses to Restricted Access* (Washington, D.C.: 1990).

On feminist movement activity on abortion in the 1960s and early 1970s, see Petchesky, *Abortion and Woman's Choice*, pp. 125–32, and Lucinda Cisler, "Unfinished Business: Birth Control and Women's Liberation," in Robin Morgan, ed., *Sisterhood Is Powerful* (New York: Vintage, 1970), pp. 245–89. Feminist actions of this period included many speak-outs, demonstrations, and – doubtless discomforting to many physicians, even those sympathetic to abortion – disruptions of both medical meetings, such as the AMA annual convention in 1970, and courtrooms which were hearing abortion-related cases. Three feminist lawyers involved in abortion litigation recalled the atmosphere in a courtroom in 1969: "One of the first instances of a courtroom demonstration by women was in connection with *Abramowitz v. Lefkowitz* [an early abortion rights case]. It was a fun demonstration, something other movements have been using right along. A substantial number of women came to court and brought two things with them: babies, crying babies, and coat hangers. When they left, they took the babies with them but left the coat hangers scattered all over the courtroom." Janice Goodman, Rhonda Copelon (Schoenbrod), and Nancy Stearns, "*Doe* and *Roe*: Where Do We Go from Here?" *Women's Rights Law Reporter* 1 (1973): 24.

Another significant feminist activity was the actual provision of illegal abortions by a group from the Chicago Women's Liberation Union, known collectively as "Jane." The group was initially established as a counseling and referral service but ultimately decided to do abortions themselves after learning techniques from one of their "doctors" who, it turned out, was a layman himself. In several years of operating, and providing approximately 3500 abortions per year, the group had no fatalities and only one encounter with the law. Garrow, *Liberty and Privacy*, pp. 486–87. See also Pauline Bart, "Seizing the Means of Reproduction: An Illegal Feminist Abortion Collective – How and Why It Worked," *Qualitative Sociology* 10 (1987): 339–57, and

"Just Call Jane," in Marlene G. Fried, ed., *From Abortion to Reproductive Freedom* (Boston: South End Press, 1990), pp. 93–100.

26. Calderone, ed., *Abortion in the United States*, pp. 58–70. At the conference, Timanus mentioned that over the course of his career, he had received abortion referrals from 353 physicians in the Washington-Baltimore area. In a somewhat subdued manner at the conference, and elsewhere more directly, Timanus expressed considerable bitterness that not one of these referring physicians answered his plea to come forward to speak on his behalf when he was tried for illegal abortion in 1950 (and subsequently served several months in prison). Calderone, ed., *Abortion in the United States*, p. 71. See also the profile of Timanus, "The Skilled Abortionist," in Lader, *Abortion*, pp. 42–51.

Edgar Keemer, an African-American physician based in Detroit, was another well-known and medically respected provider of illegal abortion in the pre-*Roe* era who drew personal satisfaction from Guttmacher's support. In his memoirs, Keemer speaks of writing in 1959 to Guttmacher from his prison cell, after being convicted of performing an illegal abortion, and of the encouraging reply he received. Keemer resumed his abortion work after his release and ultimately became a major referral point for the Clergy Consultation Service. Keemer, who was strongly committed to both the socialist and the civil rights movements, also noted approvingly in his book Guttmacher's sensitivity to the higher death rate faced by black women from illegal abortions. Edgar Keemer, *Confessions of a Pro-life Abortionist* (Detroit: Vinco Press, 1980), pp. 163–64, 214–15.

27. For various discussions of Spencer, see "Dr. Spencer," "*Commonwealth vs. Spencer*," and "Mrs. Spencer," in Patricia Miller, *The Worst of Times* (New York: Harper Collins, 1993), pp. 122–39; Lader, "The Skilled Abortionist," in *Abortion*, pp. 42–51; Michael T. Kaufman, "Abortion Doctor," *Lear's*, July–August 1989, pp. 84–87. Garrow, *Liberty and Privacy*, p. 363, reports on the extensive media coverage at the time of Spencer's death, including a lengthy obituary in the *New York Times*.

28. Robert Spencer, "The Performance of Nonhospital Abortions," in Robert Hall, ed., *Abortion in a Changing World*, vol. 1, pp. 218–25.

29. Nonetheless, several observers report that Timanus's appearance at the 1955 Planned Parenthood meeting "created much tension," in spite of Guttmacher's sponsorship. As the authors put it, "the disdain [of mainstream physicians for illegal abortionists] was painfully clear." Frederick Jaffe, Barbara Lindheim, and Philip Lee, *Abortion Politics: Private Morality and Public Policy* (New York: McGraw Hill, 1981), p. 64. Arlene Carmen and Howard Moody, the founders of the Clergy Consultation Service, noted a similar stig-

matization of physician providers of illegal abortion some fifteen years later, in the late 1960s, in *Abortion Counseling and Social Change*: "The attitude of doctors toward those persons in the profession who became 'abortionists' was one of absolute contempt. This attitude was held even by those doctors who were 'liberal' enough to refer wealthy patients to them" (p. 17).

30. Franc Novak, "Experience with Suction Curettage," in Robert Hall, ed., *Abortion in a Changing World*, vol. 1, pp. 74–84.

31. Personal communication, Helen Colvard (secretary to Lalor Burdick), March 17, 1988.

32. "Abortion and Womankind," pp. 193–209 in Hall, ed., *Abortion in a Changing World*, vol. 2. One of the participants at that session has told me that a number of women present began to speak spontaneously about their own illegal abortions.

33. Chesler, *Woman of Valor*, p. 461. The internationalization of Planned Parenthood efforts and the deepening interests of the U.S. government and private foundations in population programs after World War II have led many to point to the eugenic, often explicitly racist, motivations that often drove such efforts, a point made especially forcefully by Gordon in *Woman's Body, Woman's Right*. At the same time, international family planning efforts have long interested feminist health workers, who, while decrying the eugenic motivations of "population controllers," have nonetheless seen reproductive health services as crucial to the well-being of women in the developing world. With respect to the sensibility that drew many of the physicians interviewed in this study to international work, I would argue that in most cases it was neither a feminist vision of reproductive freedom (though sometimes this developed as a result of this work) nor heavy-handed eugenics, but rather a profound interest in public health, driven especially by the realization of the high rates of maternal and infant mortality and morbidity in the developing world.

For recent statements which attempt to bridge the longstanding gap between the feminist and public health approaches to international family planning efforts, see Ruth Dixon-Mueller, *Population Policy and Women's Rights* (Westport, Conn.: Praeger, 1993); Judith Bruce, "Users' Perspectives on Contraceptive Technology and Delivery Systems: Highlighting Some Feminist Issues," *Technology and Society* 9: 359–83; and Deborah Rogow, "Women's Health Policy: Where Lie the Interests of Physicians?" *International Journal of Gynecology and Obstetrics* 46 (1994): 237–43.

34. On the role of early feminist health activists in developing techniques

of menstrual extraction in the 1970s, see "The Development of Menstrual Extraction," in Rebecca Chalker and Carol Downer, *A Woman's Book of Choices: Abortion, Menstrual Extraction, RU-486* (New York: Four Walls, Eight Windows, 1992), pp. 113–27. For a discussion of contemporary usage of this method, see Ruth Dixon-Mueller, "Innovations in Reproductive Health Care: Menstrual Regulation Policies and Programs in Bangladesh," *Studies in Family Planning* 19 (1988): 129–40.

35. Malcolm Potts, Peter Diggory, and John Peel, *Abortion* (London: Cambridge University Press, 1977), pp. 184–45, 190, 194. See also Hodgson, ed., *Abortion and Sterilization*, pp. 213, 231, 244. See also the discussion in this volume, chapter 5, for an account of one physician's encounter with Karman.

36. Reimer (Ray) Ravenholt, the AID official who convened the 1972 Hawaii meeting, also attended the 1968 Hot Springs conference on abortion. At that occasion he said, "As Director of Population for the Agency for International Development, I am concerned with developing as rapidly as possible a program of assistance to the family-planning programs of the developing countries. I firmly believe that abortion will play a very important role in these programs." Quoted in Hall, ed., *Abortion in a Changing World*, vol. 2, p. 49.

37. Quoted in Petchesky, *Abortion and Women's Choice*, p. 124.

38. On the feminist health movement generally of the 1960s and 1970s, see Sheryl Ruzek, *The Women's Health Movement: Feminist Alternatives to Medical Control* (New York: Praeger, 1978); and Claudia Dreifus, ed., *Seizing Our Bodies: The Politics of Women's Health* (New York: Vintage, 1977). Three books that appeared during this period that were highly critical of then-prevailing obstetrical and gynecological practice were Ellen Frankfurt, *Vaginal Politics* (New York: Quadrangle Books, 1972); Barbara Seaman, *The Doctor's Case Against the Pill* (New York: Avon, 1969); and, in 1969, the first edition of the now-classic *Our Bodies, Our Selves*, perhaps the best-known (and certainly most enduring) document of the women's health movement which emerged in the 1960s. The most recent edition is published as The Boston Women's Health Book Collective, *The New Our Bodies, Our Selves* (New York: Simon and Schuster, 1992).

39. Jaffe *et al.*, *Abortion Politics*, p. 67.

40. "A Statement on Abortion by One Hundred Professors of Obstetrics," *American Journal of Obstetrics and Gynecology* 112 (1972): 992–98.

41. Hall, ed., *Abortion in a Changing World*, vol. 2, p. 108.

42. *Ibid.*, p. 108.

43. On hospital-based abortions in 1977, see Jaffe *et al.*, *Abortion Politics*, p. 32.

44. Barbara Lindheim and M. A. Cotterill, "Training in Induced Abortion by Obstetrics and Gynecology Residency Programs," *Family Planning Perspectives* 10 (1978): 24.

45. Jonathan Imber, *Abortion and the Private Practice of Medicine* (New Haven: Yale, 1986), p. 14.

46. Constance A. Nathanson and Marshall H. Becker, "The Influence of Physicians' Attitudes on Abortion Performance, Patient Management and Professional Fees," *Family Planning Perspectives* 9 (1977): 158–63.

47. Constance A. Nathanson and Marshall H. Becker, "Obstetricians' Attitudes and Hospital Abortion Services," *Family Planning Perspectives* 12 (1980): 26–32.

48. Quoted in Jaffe *et al.*, *Abortion Politics*, p. 66.

49. *Ibid.*, pp. 46–47. However, just a few years earlier, at its 1970 annual convention, the AMA House of Delegates passed a resolution endorsing abortion in either "hospitals or approved clinics." Quoted in Gerald Rosenberg, *The Hollow Hope: Can Courts Bring About Social Change?* (Chicago: University of Chicago Press, 1991), p. 199.

50. *Ibid.*, p. 45.

51. Writing in the spring of 1973, several months after the *Roe* decision, John Knowles, M.D., president of the Rockefeller Foundation and former general director of the Massachusetts General Hospital, said, "The Court's ruling mandates that government and the health system respond affirmatively with a concrete program to ensure that individuals are able to gain access to abortions performed under the safest, most dignified and most humane conditions." Knowles went on to detail the steps necessary to ensure that as many abortions as possible take place in the first trimester of pregnancy and that abortions be made available wherever the only hospitals in the area have religious objections to performing the procedure. Without such proactive efforts on the part of the medical community, Knowles predicted – correctly, as it turned out – that it would be especially difficult for the young and the poor, especially the rural poor, to obtain abortions. "The Health System and the Supreme Court Decision: An Affirmative Response," *Family Planning Perspectives* 5 (1973): 113–16.

52. Philip Darney, "Training Physicians in Elective Abortion Technique in the United States," in U. Landy and S. Ratnam, eds., *Prevention and Treatment of Contraceptive Failure* (New York: Plenum, 1986), pp. 133–40.

53. *Harris v. McCrae.* For an account of how the abortion issue preoccupied the Carter administration, see the memoir by Joseph Califano, Carter's Secretary of Health and Human Services, *Governing America* (New York: Simon and Schuster, 1981).

54. A lively account of the extreme politicization of the abortion issue, including the "gag rule" controversy, during the Reagan-Bush era is offered in Michelle McKeegan, *Abortion Politics: Mutiny in the Ranks of the Right* (New York: Free Press, 1992). The relationship of the abortion issue to a broader right-wing agenda is discussed in Rosalind Petchesky, "The Antiabortion Movement and the Rise of the New Right," in *Abortion and Women's Choice,* pp. 241–85. For a celebrated case of an abortion-driven appointment that backfired during the Reagan presidency, see the memoir of Everett Koop, Reagan's surgeon general, who in spite of his personal antiabortion views, "betrayed" the Reagan administration on a number of controversial issues, including AIDS education and the alleged existence of a "postabortion stress syndrome." *Koop: The Memoirs of America's Family Doctor* (New York: Random House, 1991). The extent to which abortion politics spilled over into birth control policies during this era, including teenage pregnancy prevention efforts, is discussed in Carole Joffe, "Sexual Politics and the Teenaged Pregnancy Prevention Worker," in Annette Lawson and Deborah Rhode, eds., *The Politics of Pregnancy: Adolescent Pregnancy and Public Policy* (New Haven: Yale University Press, 1993), pp. 284–300.

3. "THE LENGTHS TO WHICH WOMEN WOULD GO"

1. In their *Abortion Handbook for Responsible Women* (see chapter 2, n. 25), Phelan and Maginnis, besides giving advice on how to fabricate a hemorrhage that would resemble a miscarriage and thus lead to an authorized abortion, also suggested that pregnant women make an appointment for an IUD (intrauterine device) – the insertion of which, presumably, would interrupt the pregnancy. As IUDs were commonly inserted during women's menstrual cycles, this strategy involved simulating a period, about which the authors gave careful instructions: "About two hours before you and your 'period' must report in for loop installation, dip your well-scrubbed forefinger . . . into the blood on the raw liver and rub this bloody finger into your vaginal tract. Go way up, beyond your cervix, not just in the opening. Menstrual blood collects in the back of the vagina, so be sure and put some there to make it look authentic" (p. 147). As I will discuss later in this chapter and the next, however, the reports of various participants in this study suggest that inserting an IUD into a pregnant woman did not always result in an abortion.

2. For a review of the most common techniques of illegal abortion – both self-induced and performed by others – see Richard Schwartz, *Septic Abortion* (Philadelphia: J. B. Lippincott, 1968); Gordon Horobin, ed., *Experience with Abortion* (New York: Cambridge University Press, 1973), and Potts *et al.*, *Abortion*, pp. 253–76. For an account of the medical challenges that were involved in treating certain types of illegal abortions, see Michael Burnhill, "Treatment of Women Who Have Undergone Chemically Induced Abortions," *Journal of Reproductive Medicine* 30 (1985): 610–14.

3. Leunbach paste was also the method used for many years with apparent success by Ed Keemer, a highly regarded provider of illegal abortion in the Detroit area (see chapter 2, n. 26), *Confessions of a Pro-life Abortionist*, pp. 65–70. This paste was also extensively discussed at a 1970 San Francisco symposium on abortion, as reported in Thomas Hart, ed., *First American Symposium on Office Abortions: The Proceedings of the Symposium of Office Abortion Procedures* (San Francisco: Society for Humane Abortion, 1970).

4. This issue of opponents of abortion having a double standard for family members reached a high point of visibility during the 1992 presidential campaign, when both George Bush and his vice-presidential candidate, Dan Quayle, gave equivocal answers when questioned hypothetically about abortion as a choice made by their own family members – even though both were running on a strong antiabortion platform. Kevin Sack, "Quayle Insists Abortion Remarks Don't Signal Change in His View," *New York Times*, July 24, 1992, pp. A1, A12; Andrew Rosenthal, "Bush, Asked in Personal Context, Takes a Softer Stand on Abortion," *New York Times*, August 12, 1992, pp. A1, A15.

5. Bernard Nathanson, a physician very active in abortion reform in New York (and who later became controversial for his dramatic turnabout on the abortion issue) offers, in his memoir, a vivid account of the different condition and experiences of the clinic patient and the private abortion patient in his hospital. After outlining the typically gruesome details of the former ("bleeding profusely" at 2:00 A.M. in the emergency room, with a temperature of 103 or 104 degrees, "another victim of a hack abortionist or of self-abortion," "uncontrollable infection" that could lead to death or a hysterectomy), Nathanson writes: "A little different story with the private patients. If you were the resident on the private service, the call would usually come at seven or eight in the evening, a short time after office hours. The private physician would be on the other end of the line advising you that he was sending in Mrs. Buggins with heavy vaginal bleeding, the diagnosis being incomplete abortion – that is, miscarriage. He wanted to do the D. & C. in a couple of hours, so would you please prepare her for the O.R. and inform the anesthe-

sia people? ... She would invariably appear in an astonishingly blooming state of health and her sanitary pad would have a single dime-sized stain of blood on it. . . . She would be wheeled into the O. R. and coaxed gently to sleep by a solicitous anesthesiologist . . . Then the private physician would appear to be ceremoniously gowned and gloved for the operation." Nathanson, *Aborting America* (Garden City, N.Y.: Doubleday, 1979), pp. 19–22.

6. Roots's career is discussed in Reed, *The Birth Control Movement and American Society*, p. 299.

4. "I WAS DOING IT FOR REASONS OF CONSCIENCE"

1. A fictional account of substituting tissue to circumvent antiabortion law is Michael Crichton's *A Case of Need* (New York: Dutton, 1993). The book was originally published in 1968, with Crichton writing under the name of Jeffrey Hudson.

2. Darrow is referring to a 1985 novel by John Irving, *The Cider House Rules* (New York: William Morrow, 1985) in which the hero, a crusty but saintly country doctor who simultaneously runs an orphanage and provides obstetrical services, comes to realize the necessity of providing abortions as well.

3. Guttmacher first came to national prominence as a forceful advocate of birth control education and dissemination, writing several books for a lay audience on the subject, including *Babies by Choice or by Chance* (Garden City: Doubleday, 1959). His evolution to an abortion rights position was a gradual one, as he moved from support for abortion in limited circumstances (the ALI proposal) and under the regulated conditions of physician committee approval (a system he had initiated) to, ultimately, support for "abortion on request." As Guttmacher wrote in 1970, "From these experiences [of states which had been among the first to liberalize abortion laws] . . . I reluctantly concluded that abortion on request – necessitating removal of 'abortion' from the penal codes – was the only way to truly democratize legal abortion and to sufficiently increase the numbers performed so as to decrease the incidence of illegal abortions. I came to this conclusion in 1969, forty-seven years after abortion first came to my attention as a medical student." Guttmacher, "The Genesis of Liberalized Abortion in New York," pp. 551–52.

Though, undoubtedly, as Fieldstone's remarks suggest, Guttmacher did much to legitimate abortion practice at Mt. Sinai, one of New York's premier medical institutions, his efforts were not appreciated by all his colleagues. As a junior associate later wrote, "Many members of the staff felt that Dr. Guttmacher had breached normal medical-moral discipline by allowing abortions to be performed at the hospital." Quoted in Garrow, *Liberty and Privacy*, p. 277.

4. Fieldstone is most likely referring to a notorious incident that occurred in New York City on Christmas Eve, 1955, in which an unskilled lay abortionist, faced with the death of a patient, dismembered her body and disposed of the various pieces in trash cans along Broadway. See Lader, *Abortion*, p. 64.

5. Fieldstone is referring to Maginnis and Phelan, *The Abortion Handbook for Responsible Women*. (See chapter 2, n. 25, and chapter 3, n. 1.)

6. For an account of the founding of the CCS, see Carmen and Moody, *Abortion Counseling and Social Change*. The estimate of one hundred thousand abortion referrals without a fatality is on p. 75.

7. On Morgentaler's life generally, see Eleanor Wright Pelrine, *Morgentaler: The Doctor Who Couldn't Turn Away* (Toronto: Gage Publishing Co., 1975) and Anne Collins, *The Big Evasion: Abortion, the Issue that Won't Go Away* (Toronto: Lester and Orpen Dennys Ltd., 1985). On Morgentaler's legal battles with the Canadian government, see F. L. Morton, *Morgentaler v. Borowski: Abortion, the Charter, and the Courts* (Toronto: McClelland Stewart, 1992); A. Anne McLellan, "Abortion Law in Canada," in Butler and Walbert, *Abortion, Medicine and the Law*, pp. 333–67; and Morgentaler's own essay, "My Struggle for Abortion Rights in Canada," *Religious Humanism* 26 (1992): 159–73.

8. This comment of Morgentaler's – that he was spurred to offer illegal abortions as it became increasingly clear that other outlets for such abortions were disappearing – suggests an intriguing link between Morgentaler's behavior and recent research on altruism, especially the notion that altrustic behavior is more likely to occur if the individual feels he or she is the only one available to help in a given situation. See Jane A. Piliavin and Hong-Wen Charng, "Altruism: A Review of Recent Theory and Research," *Annual Review of Sociology* 16 (1990): 27–65, esp. p. 35. I am indebted to Ann Swidler for bringing this to my attention.

9. Morgentaler, "My Struggle for Abortion Rights," p. 162.

10. *Ibid.*, pp. 163–64.

11. *Ibid.*, pp. 164–65.

12. *Morgentaler* (1988) and its relationship to subsequent abortion cases in Canada is discussed in detail in McLellan, "Abortion Law in Canada," pp. 333–43.

13. See, for example, Joseph Fabry, Reuven Bulka, and William Sahakian, *Logotherapy* (New York: J. Aronson, 1979).

5. "I WANTED TO DO SOMETHING ABOUT ABORTION"

1. On the Belous case, and the subsequent mobilization of many in the pro-choice legal and medical communities, see Garrow, *Liberty and Privacy*, pp. 354–56, 364–66, 377–79.

2. The Society for Humane Abortion, headed by Patricia Maginnis in San Francisco, in the mid-1960s operated a referral service for abortions in Mexico, and the records of the organization make clear the ever-changing status of "reliable" clinics and individual physicians – reports of "hassle-free" and medically sound service at a particular facility would be shortly followed by warnings that an abortion at the same clinic now might involve additional payoffs to police, less competent treatment, no English-speaking personnel, and so on. See the Papers of the Society for Humane Abortion, at the Schlesinger Library, Radcliffe College, Cambridge, Mass.

3. As the founders of the Clergy Counseling Service described the organization's monitoring of physicians: "Our monitoring technique was simple and dependable since the patients themselves did it for us. When a new doctor was tentatively 'approved,' only one member of the CCS was authorized to make referrals to him. That minister or rabbi would urge every woman who saw the doctor to report back, either in person or by mail, any discrepancies between what she had been led to expect and what actually occurred. Was the medical and psychological treatment satisfactory? . . . After three or four weeks, if we received consistently satisfactory reports from the women, information about this new 'resource' would be shared with all of the other members of the CCS. . . . A surprisingly high percentage (40 percent) of all counselees did recontact their counselor after the abortion, providing us with a steady stream of information about the doctors we were using." Carmen and Moody, *Abortion Counseling and Social Change*, p. 43.

4. As Bates and Zawadzki stated in *Criminal Abortion*, in summarizing the prevailing legal situation during the 1950s and 1960s: "Any person who assists in an abortion procedure is equally guilty as the person who manipulates instruments or administers any drug or substance. A conviction for the crime of abortion was obtained even though it was shown that the physician in question did not handle the instruments himself. The fact that he aided and assisted was no less criminal than the actual manipulation of the instruments" (pp. 104–5).

5. In "The Genesis of Liberalized Abortion in New York," Guttmacher reflects on his eventual disillusionment with "reform" approaches to abortion and his embrace of the more radical "abortion on request" position, citing the imperfect workings of the psychiatric consultations as a prime factor in his

change of heart: "I examined the situation personally in Colorado and discovered that two Denver hospitals were doing virtually all of the pregnancy
interruptions and these were being performed primarily on the private sec-
tor. This clearly implied that the state-imposed requirement of two psychiatric consultations was causing an effective discrimination against ward patients: private consultations were too expensive as to be available only to the
wealthier patients, and psychiatric appointments in public facilities were
booked solid for three months – far beyond the time limitation on obtaining
an abortion" (p. 552).

Solinger, in examining the discussion of psychiatric indications for abortion that took place in medical journals in the 1950s and 1960s, found a deep
uneasiness among many ob/gyns about involving psychiatrists in medical
decisions. As she wrote, "Many . . . were most concerned that the use of psychiatric findings in favor of abortion further undermined the traditions and
the reputation of medicine as a scientific endeavor. Psychiatry was merely a
'long practiced art,' at best 'an infant science.'" Solinger, "'A Complete Disaster': Abortion and the Politics of Hospital Abortion Committees, 1950–1970,"
Feminist Studies 19 (1993): 248.

6. Richard Lamm, as a novice Colorado state legislator in 1967, introduced
an abortion reform bill (based on the ALI proposal) that became the first
such bill to pass in a state legislature. Lamm's career as an abortion rights
advocate – and his fairly rapid disavowal of such limited reform efforts – are
discussed in Garrow, *Liberty and Privacy*, pp. 323–25, 327, 329, 383–84, 482,
485.

7. On the opening of the CCS facility, see Carmen and Moody, *Abortion
Counseling and Social Change*, pp. 67–82. However, not all within the medical
community – even those supportive of abortion – were persuaded of the
safety of freestanding clinics. Besides the 1970 AMA resolution which had
called for abortions to take place only in hospitals, the New York City Health
Department and the New York Academy of Medicine also argued against
abortions taking place in clinics. Robert Hall – who had been the founder of
the Association for Humane Abortion – was perhaps the most prominent pro-
choice physician who initially spoke out strongly against the freestanding
clinics, also on safety grounds. Hall's opposition to clinics, however, was also
based on his fears that such a development would facilitate the evasion of
abortion on the part of hospitals. Speaking in 1970, in a statement that has
proved remarkably prophetic, Hall said, "I want to see the hospitals forced to
perform abortions. If we let them off the hook by setting up clinics, they'll
never accept their responsibilities." Quoted in Garrow, *Liberty and Privacy*,
p. 456.

8. Immediately after the 1970 repeal in New York state, a number of referral services tailored to out-of-town abortion patients were established. Some of these were nonprofit and affiliated with various feminist groups, others were commercial referral services. The latter were shortly banned by law. Garrow, *Liberty and Privacy*, p. 494.

9. On the principles of abortion counseling, see Terry Beresford, *Short Term Relationship Counseling*, 2d ed. (Baltimore, Md.: Planned Parenthood of Maryland, 1988). On the early political roots of abortion counseling, and the new occupation's subsequent evolution into a more conventional role within a medicalized hierarchy, see Carole Joffe, *The Regulation of Sexuality: Experiences of Family Planning Workers* (Philadelphia: Temple University Press, 1986).

10. Recollecting the atmosphere in one of the first abortion clinics to open in New York, a former counselor – in terms quite similar to Fieldstone's – captured both the sense of colleagueship *and* tension that existed then between counselors and physicians: "It blows my mind, thinking about it now, about how much power we [the counselors] had. . . . The doctors were just terribly nervous about the whole thing and were willing to listen to us – about what kind of counseling services there should be, lots of things. If one of the doctors they hired was causing too much pain or saying disgusting things to patients, we'd run into the director's office and get him fired. Unfortunately, the honeymoon period didn't last long though." Quoted in Joffe, *The Regulation of Sexuality*, p. 36.

11. On the use of the paracervical block in freestanding clinics, see Jane Hodgson, ed., *Abortion and Sterilization*, pp. 241–44, 257, 523; and Warren Hern, *Abortion Practice* (Philadelphia: J. B. Lippincott, 1984), pp. 113–14.

12. Lader, *Abortion II*, pp. 113–14; on the Gesell ruling, see Garrow, *Liberty and Privacy*, pp. 382, 383, 386, 407.

13. Christopher Tietze and Sarah Lewit, "Joint Program for the Study of Abortions," *Studies in Family Planning* 3 (1972): 97–124.

14. As I discuss in chapter 7, such waiting periods – which are now legislatively mandated in a number of states – are strongly opposed by most abortion providers, because of the hardships they impose on abortion recipients, especially those who must travel a long way to an abortion clinic.

6. "GETTING YOUR HANDS DIRTY"

1. *Roe v. Wade*, 410 U.S. 113 (1973). It was actually the companion case to *Roe– Doe v. Bolton*, 410 U.S. 179 (1973) – that facilitated the freestanding clinic,

by expressly stating that abortions did not have to be restricted to hospitals. The analysis of the political scientist Gerald Rosenberg is that abortion reformers "got very lucky" in that it was Justice Harry Blackmun, the author of the *Doe* (as well as the *Roe*) opinion, who was largely responsible for this provision, as the original briefs had made minimal mention of the setting where abortions could be performed. Gerald N. Rosenberg, *The Hollow Hope: Can Courts Bring About Social Change?* (Chicago: University of Chicago Press, 1991), chap. 6, pp. 175–202.

2. As two public health physicians point out, "Because abortion has been so controversial, it has been highly scrutinized, and the *health benefits* to women are incontrovertible." Wendy Chavkin and Allan Rosenfeld, "Reply to J. Wilke," *American Journal of Obstetrics and Gynecology* 167 (1992): 855, emphasis theirs. The improvement in death and complication rates became immediately apparent after the legalization of abortion. As Ward Cates, formerly head of the Abortion Surveillance Unit at the Center for Disease Control, wrote: "The decline of abortion mortality rapidly accelerated in 1970 and generally continued through 1976. . . . This accelerated decline further suggests that legal abortions were primarily replacing illegal abortions. . . . The increase in physician training and experience may be one factor . . . in the decrease in deaths related to induced abortion after 1975. . . . The death-to-case rate for legal abortion has decreased from 6.2 per 100,000 in 1970 to 1.5 in 1979. Improvements in anesthesia technique, use of better methods of dilation, reductions in the use of hysterotomy or hysterectomy for purposes of abortion, greater willingness to reevacuate a uterus if retained tissue is suspected, and physicians' familiarity with other abortion complications all may have contributed." Ward Cates, "Legal Abortion: The Public Health Record," *Science* 215 (1982): 1586–87. See also Council on Scientific Affairs, "Induced Termination of Pregnancy Before and After *Roe v. Wade*: Trends in the Mortality and Morbidity of Women," *Journal of the American Medical Association* 268 (1992): 3231–39.

3. Hodgson, ed., *Abortion and Sterilization*, pp. 522–23.

4. See Judith Bourne, "Influences on Health Professionals' Attitudes Towards Abortion," *Journal of the American Hospital Association* 46 (1972): 80–83; F. J. Kane *et al.*, "Emotional Reactions in Abortion Services Personnel," *Archives of General Psychiatry* 28 (1973): 409–11; Howard D. Kibel, "Staff Reactions to Abortion," *Obstetrics and Gynecology* 39 (1972): 128–33; and, especially, Marianne Such-Baer, "Professional Staff Reaction to Abortion Work," *Social Casework* 55 (1974): 435–41.

5. See, for example, Warren Hern and Bonnie Andrikopoulos, eds., *Abortion in the Seventies: Proceedings of the Western Regional Conference on Abor-*

tion (New York: National Abortion Federation, 1977). The published proceedings of this conference, which was held in Denver in 1976, are noteworthy for opening with a letter of "warmest greetings" from then First Lady Betty Ford – a sharp contrast to the subsequent politics of abortion within the Republican party, as evidenced by the admission of pro-choice sympathies by two former First Ladies (Barbara Bush and Nancy Reagan) that came only after their husbands left office.

6. John Westfall, Ken Kallail, and Anne Walling, "Abortion Attitudes and Practices of Family and General Practice Physicians," *The Journal of Family Practice* 33 (1991): 47–91. In their survey of family practitioners in Kansas, the authors found that while only 56 percent of those in their survey reported themselves as "pro-choice," 78 percent of the respondents believed that abortion should be legal (while 8 percent believed it should not be legal), and that 77 percent of the survey group had referred a woman for an abortion within the past year (p. 48). In a survey of its membership in 1985, the American College of Obstetricians and Gynecologists found that of those members who did "not believe abortion should ever be performed (13 percent of the total responding), 55 percent said they would refer a woman to an abortion provider." "ACOG Poll: Ob-Gyns' Support for Abortion Unchanged Since 1971," *Family Planning Perspectives* 17 (1985): 275.

7. Writing about the management of complications that had occurred within a population of twenty thousand women receiving first trimester abortions at Preterm in Washington in the early 1970s, just before *Roe*, Jane Hodgson spoke of the problem of "fragmented care" – those women experiencing complications had returned to their hometowns where they had to deal with a medical establishment often unfamiliar with abortion care and hostile to abortion, as well. Reviewing the hospital records and pathological reports, Hodgson concluded that in the case of the most common complication – tissue retention – a number of hospitalizations for a D. & C. (rather than the far simpler reevacuation of the uterus) "may have been unnecessary, even punitive." She similarly found cases of questionable sterilizations occurring in response to complications, as well as unnecessary laparotomies. Writing this article shortly after the *Roe* decision was announced, Hodgson voiced hope that "complication rates can be further lowered by elimination of fragmented abortion care. With uniform legalization of abortion throughout our 50 states, the profession should dispose of this problem and provide the patient who has an unwanted pregnancy with continuous, humane, and high-quality care, preferably administered by a single physician or group of physicians." Jane Hodgson, "Major Complications of 20,248 Consecutive First Trimester Abortions: Problems of Fragmented Care," *Advances in Planned Parenthood* IX (1975): 52–59.

Yet, given that abortion services are currently only available in 16 percent of U.S. counties, today many of those abortion recipients with complications still must receive postabortion care from physicians different from those who performed the procedure, and, according to the accounts of Hodgson and others, continue to be vulnerable to medical overreaction and reprisal.

8. On malpractice issues facing ob/gyns, see Mark Taragin, Adam Wilczek, Elizabeth Karns, Richard Trout, and Jeffrey Carson, "Physician Demographics and the Risk of Malpractice," *The American Journal of Medicine* 93 (1992): 537–42, which states, "Specialty was strongly associated with claims rate, with neurosurgery, orthopedics, and obstetrics/gynecology having 7–12 times the number of claims per year as psychiatry, the specialty with the fewest claims" (p. 537). See also J. F. Hough and M. W. Jones, "Professional Liability Issues in Obstetrical Practice," *Socioeconomic Report of the California Medical Association* 25 (1985): 1–4, which reports both on a "burgeoning incidence of malpractice litigation involving obstetrical events" and a "steady escalation of premiums for professional liability coverage" (p. 1). The rise of specialized law firms, affiliated with the antiabortion movement, to prosecute abortion-related claims is discussed in the next chapter.

9. Stanley Henshaw and Jennifer Van Vort, "Abortion Services in the United States, 1991–92," *Family Planning Perspectives* 26 (1994), p. 100.

10. David Grimes, Jacqueline Forrest, Alice Kirkman, and Barbara Radford, "An Epidemic of Antiabortion Violence in the United States," *American Journal of Obstetrics and Gynecology* 165 (1991): 1263–68. The emergence of the violent wing of the antiabortion movement is chronicled in Dallas Blanchard and Terry Prewitt, *Religious Violence and Abortion: The Gideon Project* (Gainesville: University of Florida Press, 1993), and Dallas Blanchard, *The Antiabortion Movement and the Rise of the Religious Right.* See also Barbara Radford and Gina Shaw, "Antiabortion Violence: Causes and Effects," *Women's Health Issues* 3 (1993): 144–51.

11. As Henshaw and Van Vort report in their *Abortion Factbook*, "Over half the providers of 400 or more abortions a year report having been picketed at least 20 times during the year; many of these providers face weekly or even daily picketing. Almost half report picketing with physical contact or blocking of patients, and more than one third have been the site of at least one demonstration resulting in arrests" (p. 54).

A clinic director in a suburban location related an interesting incident of at least momentary solidarity between picketers and clinic staff. The director was called by the local police, who had received a report that someone had entered a clinic with a gun. The police came to the clinic and apprehended a man with a gun in the clinic waiting room who turned out to be an off-duty security guard accompanying his wife for her abortion. They later found out that the police had initially been notified by the "regular" picketers outside the clinic, who did not want to take the blame for any violence that might ensue.

12. In a small number of communities, activists on both sides of the abortion issue have attempted dialogue and some joint projects, under the name of "Common Ground." The first such effort, and the best known to date, has taken place in St. Louis, where the group has worked together on issues such as adoption, better prenatal care, aid to pregnant women who are drug-addicted, and prevention of unwanted pregnancy. See Tamar Lewin, "In Bitter Abortion Debate, Opponents Learn to Reach for Common Ground," *New York Times*, February 17, 1992, p. A7. A more tenuous "common ground" effort that took place in North Dakota is described in Faye Ginsburg, *Contested Lives: The Abortion Debate in an American Community* (Berkeley: University of California Press, 1989).

13. The activities of "abortion entrepreneurs" and especially the streamlining of abortion procedures in certain types of for-profit clinics are described in two articles by Michael Goldstein about the creation of an "abortion market" in Southern California: "Creating and Controlling a Medical Market: Abortion in Los Angeles After Liberalization," *Social Problems* 31 (1984): 414–529, and "Abortion as a Medical Career Choice: Entrepreneurs, Community Physicians, and Others," *Journal of Health and Social Behavior* 25 (1984): 211–29. Goldstein (in "Creating and Controlling a Medical Market," p. 527) makes the interesting point that some among those he studied conceived of themselves as "entrepreneurs" (that is, perceived medicine primarily in terms of economic opportunity) before entering abortion work, while for others, the stigmatization by other physicians that they felt as abortion providers in itself facilitated an "entrepreneurial" identity.

14. Some nurses find assisting at saline abortions, a common technique of second trimester abortion during the period Phillips is referring to, more emotionally difficult than other types of abortion. After the pregnant woman has had saline solution injected into her amniotic sac, nurses are obliged to monitor her for about twenty-four to thirty-six hours until she eventually expels the dead fetus. See Thomas D. Kerenyi, "Intraamniotic techniques," in J. Hodgson, ed., *Abortion and Sterilization: Medical and Social Aspects* (New York: Grune and Stratton, 1981), pp. 359–77.

15. Blanchard writes in *The Antiabortion Movement and the Rise of the Religious Right* that in the course of contacting all freestanding abortion

facilities that had been the target of antiabortion violence prior to 1991, "A representative of *every* such clinic reported that at least one former picketer had later come seeking an abortion for herself or her daughter" (p. 130, emphasis his). On antiabortionists receiving abortions, see also Luker, *Abortion and the Politics of Motherhood*, pp. 174–75, and Adrienne Fugh-Berman, "Right to Lifers Learn Facts of Life," *Off Our Backs*, June 1981, p. 4.

16. On the dismal status of current contraceptive research in the United States, see the report issued by the National Research Council, Institute of Medicine, *Developing New Contraceptives: Obstacles and Opportunities*, ed. Luigi Mastroianni, Peter Donaldson, and Thomas Kane (Washington, D.C.: National Academy Press, 1990).

17. The 54 percent figure on unintended pregnancies cited by Fieldstone is found in Jacqueline Forrest, "Unintended Pregnancy Among American Women," *Family Planning Perspectives* 19 (1987): 76–77.

7. ASSURING A FUTURE FOR LEGAL ABORTION

1. Additionally, of course, the outcomes of national elections have a tremendous ability to affect abortion services. As of this writing, in the immediate aftermath of decisive Republican victories in the fall 1994 election, which resulted in Republican control of both the House and Senate (and considerably more antiabortion votes added to each chamber, especially the House), the implications for abortion provision are not entirely clear, but are nonetheless worrisome. In sharp contrast to the 1992 election, and in tacit recognition that its previously extreme antiabortion position had been costly, the Republican party as a whole downplayed its opposition to abortion in 1994, and abortion *per se* was an overt factor in very few races. Most observers agree that antiabortion forces will not, in the short run at least, attempt an outright statutory ban on abortion, but rather will "chip away" at the various gains made during the first years of the Clinton presidency. For example, the "Contract with America," put forward during the election by Republicans, calls for the restoration of the "gag rule" on abortion counseling in federally supported family planning clinics that had initially been put in place during the Reagan-Bush years and was then overturned by President Clinton (see chapter 2). Most ominous, however, from the point of view of providers, is the probable withdrawal of aggressive federal protection of clinics – for example, the posting of federal marshals at clinics that took place after the summer 1994 murders of John Britton and James Barrett. As one reporter wrote immediately after the election, "And while the law guaranteeing access to abortion clinics isn't likely to be challenged, it may be 'cleaned up,' according to a

Republican official. 'We can do that without alienating the public,' the official added." Fred Barnes, "Life of the Party," *The New Republic*, December 5, 1994, p. 10.

To be sure, even before the Republican takeover of Congress in the aftermath of the 1994 election, abortion providers were concerned about the depth of the federal commitment to protect clinics. In August 1994, there were federal marshals at twenty-five clinics in eighteen cities; by December 1994, the Justice Department, pointing to limited resources, was supplying marshals at only twelve clinics in ten cities. Tamar Lewin, "Abortion Providers Attempt to Handle Growing Threat," *New York Times*, December 31, 1994, p. A8.

2. Kitty Kolbert and Andrea Miller, "Government in the Examining Room: Restrictions on the Provision of Abortion," *Journal of the American Medical Women's Association* 49 (1994): 153–55, 164.

3. Eve Paul, "Letter to the Editor," *New York Times*, Sept. 30, 1993, p. A22.

4. As Terry Beresford, a leading trainer of abortion counselors, has written in *Short Term Relationship Counseling*, "The counselor uses the tools of active listening, attending, paraphrasing, reflecting feelings, open questioning and summarizing to facilitate a flow of information, both feeling and factual. Her effective use of these skills depends upon the client's ability to communicate and willingness to introspect. Together they facilitate the successful unfolding of the counseling relationship" (p. 108).

5. Center for Reproductive Law and Policy, "An Analysis of *Planned Parenthood v. Casey*," *Reproductive Freedom in Focus*, New York, 1992, p. 7.

6. Henshaw and Van Vort, *Abortion Factbook*, p. 179.

7. Kolbert and Miller, "Government in the Examining Room," p. 154. Besides resulting in more second trimester abortions, Althaus and Henshaw conclude that mandatory delay laws in Mississippi also "prevented approximately 11–13 percent of the women who would have had abortions from doing so.... Some women may mistakenly believe that abortion services are no longer available or are more difficult to obtain than is in fact the case. This would explain the disproportionate effect on women without a high school education." Frances Althaus and Stanley Henshaw, "The Effects of Mandatory Delay Laws on Abortion Patients and Providers," *Family Planning Perspectives* 26 (1994): 228–31, 233, at p. 233.

8. Both Michael Griffin, who killed David Gunn, and Paul Hill, who killed John Britton and James Barrett, were subsequently convicted and sentenced to life sentences. Hill, who also received a death sentence in a Florida state court, was additionally prosecuted under the new FACE legislation. Michael

Wines, "Senate Approves Bill to Protect Abortion Clinics," *New York Times*, May 13, 1994, pp. A1, A12; David Johnston, "Federal Agents Sent to Protect Abortion Clinics," *New York Times*, August 2, 1994, pp. A1, A10; *ibid.*, "F.B.I. Undertakes Conspiracy Inquiry in Clinic Violence," *New York Times*, August 4, 1994, pp. A1, A7; Bob Ortega, "Stalking Laws Used to Fight Abortion Foes," *Wall Street Journal*, April 7, 1993, pp. B1, B10; "Driver I.D. at Clinics Protected," *Washington Memo* (New York: Alan Guttmacher Institute), August 31, 1994, p. 6; *Madsen v. Women's Health Center, Inc.*, U.S. 114 SCt 2516. *Madsen* was only a partial victory for the abortion rights movement in that the Court struck down a three-hundred-foot buffer zone around the clinic and around the homes of clinic physicians and other staff. The Court, however, indicated that a smaller zone or restrictions on the size and duration of demonstrations at providers' homes might be found constitutional. Linda Greenhouse, "High Court Backs Limits on Protest at Abortion Clinic," *New York Times*, July 1, 1994, pp. A1, A9.

9. After David Gunn was murdered, a petition was circulated within anti-abortion circles that declared Gunn's death "justifiable" and stated the "justice of taking all godly action necessary to defend human life, including the use of force." The petition was circulated by Paul Hill, who later was convicted for the murders of John Britton and James Barrett, and was signed by over thirty well-known figures in the extremist wing of the antiabortion movement. The Britton-Barrett murders, and Hill's conviction, were followed by yet another declaration of the justification of such murders by various signers of the petition. See Lisa Belkin, "Kill for Life?" *New York Times Magazine*, October 30, 1994, pp. 47–51, 62–64, 76, 80; "Abortion: Who's Behind the Violence?" *U.S. News and World Report*, November 14, 1994, pp. 50–67; and Gustav Niebuhr, "To Church's Dismay, Priest Talks of 'Justifiable Homicide,'" *New York Times*, August 24, 1994, p. A12.

10. For example, in 1989 there were 201 incidents of clinic blockades, resulting in over 12,000 arrests, while in 1994, there were just 25 such incidents, resulting in 217 arrests. Yet in terms of those activities categorized by the National Abortion Federation as "violent" (murder, attempted murder, bombing, firebombing, arson, assault and battery, etc.), there were 76 such incidents in 1989, and 159 in 1994. National Abortion Federation, Washington, D.C., February 1995, "Incidents of Violence and Disruption Against Abortion Providers, 1994."

11. Garrow, *Liberty and Privacy*, pp. 688–89. George Bush also demoralized abortion providers by his statement during the 1988 presidential campaign that doctors who provide abortions should be imprisoned. This state-

ment actually was delivered as a "clarification" the morning after a debate
with his Democratic opponent, Michael Dukakis, in which Bush acknowledged he had not yet "sorted out" the penalties to be imposed if abortion were
made illegal. After an emergency late-night session of his advisers, his campaign chairman announced the following morning that Bush did not want to
be understood as advocating punishment for women who seek abortions, the
"additional victims" (in Bush's view) of the abortion, but felt punishment
should be properly directed at abortion providers. Gerald Boyd, "Bush Camp
Offers a Clarified Stand About Abortions," *New York Times*, September 27,
1988, pp. A1, B7.

12. A television commercial produced by the antiabortion group Life Dynamics, and made available to abortion malpractice lawyers, shows a dis-
tressed woman on a stormy night, with a voice-over saying, "If you've been
physically or emotionally injured by an abortion, don't suffer in silence. You
have a right to seek compensation in a court of law." Junda Woo, "Abortion
Doctors' Patients Broaden Suits," *Wall Street Journal*, October 28, 1964, p. B12.
See also Julie Cohen, "Protecting Women or Harassing Doctors? New Malpractice Firm Wades into Abortion Battle," *Legal Times*, February 14, 1994,
pp. 1, 22–23.

13. Allan Rosenfeld, "RU 486," editorial, *American Journal of Public
Health* 82 (1992): 1325–26.

14. Suzanna Banwell and John Paxman, "The Search for Meaning: RU
486 and the Law of Abortion," *American Journal of Public Health* 82 (1992):
1399.

15. Mary Ann Castle and Francine Coetaux, "RU 486 Beyond the Controversy: Implications for Health Care Practice," *Journal of the American
Women's Medical Association* 49 (1994): 156–59, 164. When testing of the drug
began in fall 1994 at a number of Planned Parenthood and other clinics, administrators were surprised at the very strong reception, as thousands of
women began to call to volunteer to take part in trials. See Maureen Balleza,
"Many Women Eager to Test Abortion Pill," *New York Times*, November 20,
1994, p. A11.

16. Katharine Seelye, "Enter RU-486, Exit Hype," *New York Times*, May 22,
1994, p. E16.

17. Henshaw and Van Vort, *Abortion Factbook*, p. 38.

18. John Tierney, "A Lone Doctor Adapts Drugs for Abortions," *New York
Times*, October 10, 1994, pp. A1, B12. See also Mitchell Creinen and Philip Darney, "Methotrexate and Misoprostol for Early Abortion," *Contraception* 48

(1993): 339–48, for one of the first reports of clinical trials of this regime. In Brazil, where abortion is illegal under most circumstances, Cytotec (the commercial name for misoprostol) has been widely used to induce abortion. Regina Barbosa and Margareth Arilha, "The Brazilian Experience with Cytotec," *Studies in Family Planning* 24 (1993): 236–40.

Yet another means of preventing pregnancy – which some argue would significantly cut down on the number of abortions if used more aggressively, is "postcoital hormonal contraception," a prescribed dosage of a combined estrogen-progestin pill, which either prevents fertilization or stops the fertilized egg from implanting. Sometimes also referred to as "the morning after pill" (though effective up to seventy-two hours after intercourse) and more recently as "emergency oral contraception," this treatment has long been offered to rape victims, but – although legal – has not been widely available to the general public. See James Trussell and Felicia Stewart, "The Effectiveness of Postcoital Hormonal Contraception," *Family Planning Perspectives* 24 (1992): 262–64. The authors contend that if this treatment were more widely available, unintended pregnancies in the United States could be reduced by as much as 1.7 million annually, and the number of abortions could be reduced by 800,000. See also Jan Hoffman, "The Morning After Pill: A Well-Kept Secret," *New York Times Magazine*, January 10, 1993, pp. 12–15, 30, 32.

In November 1994, the American Public Health Association, the American Women's Medical Association, and Planned Parenthood of New York City filed a petition with the Food and Drug Administration (FDA), urging the agency to require relabeling of six oral contraceptives as appropriate for use as morning after pills. Out of some fifty currently available brands of oral contraception in the United States, the six named in the petition have been proved effective for use as emergency postcoital contraception, and the petition claims that this information has been deliberately withheld from physicians and consumers by the manufacturers. See "Medical Groups and Health Care Providers Petition FDA to Relabel Six Oral Contraceptives as 'Morning After Pills,'" *Reproductive Freedom News*, Center for Reproductive Law and Policy, December 2, 1994, p. 4.

19. At present, the majority of private insurance plans, in fact, do cover abortion: "Sixty-six percent of fee-for-service plans, 83 percent of point of service networks, and 70 percent of HMOs routinely cover abortion services." Sharon Lerner and Janet Freedman, "Abortion and Health Care Reform," *Journal of the American Women's Medical Association* 49 (1994): 144–45, 149, at p. 144. However, because of privacy concerns, many women choose to bypass their insurance plans when obtaining an abortion.

20. Stanley Henshaw, personal communication, October 21, 1993.

21. Statement of the Independent Abortion Providers Caucus of the National Abortion Federation, April 23, 1994, Cincinnati, Ohio.

22. Michael Policar, "Health Care Reform and Abortion Services," presented at the annual meeting of the National Abortion Federation, Cincinnati, Ohio, 1994.

23. *Who Will Provide Abortions? Ensuring the Availability of Qualified Practitioners* (Washington, D.C.: National Abortion Federation, 1991).

24. The new requirement, scheduled to take effect on January 1, 1996, calls for residents to be trained in abortion procedures at the teaching hospitals where they work. Explaining the rationale for this requirement, the Accreditation Council for Graduate Medical Education pointed to concerns about the competence of doctors called upon to perform hospital-based abortions in emergency situations, in light of the fact that so few routine abortions are performed in that setting. See James Barron, "Group Requiring Abortion Study," *New York Times*, February 15, 1995, pp. A1, A10.

In addition to opt-out clauses for individual residents with moral or religious objections to abortion, the new standard also allows institutions with such objections to arrange to have their residents trained at another institution. These provisions notwithstanding, the new requirement has, predictably, generated intense opposition from Catholic medical institutions (which represent 45 of the more than 270 accredited residency programs in ob/gyn). The ACGME action also quickly drew the attention of antiabortion legislators in Congress. In what medical officials angrily denounced as unprecedented intrusion into medical accreditation activity, House and Senate legislators held hearings on the abortion training standard, and the House Appropriations Committee passed an amendment designed to nullify the new policy. As this book goes to press, in mid-1995, the eventual fate of this requirement remains unclear. See Jerry Gray, "Senate Approves Cutback in Current Federal Budget," *New York Times*, July 22, 1995, p. A7.

25. Michele Robinson, "ACOG Plan Supports Non-MD Abortions," *Ob/Gyn News*, September 1, 1994, pp. 1, 17. Additionally, in 1991, the membership of the American College of Nurse-Midwives approved a measure calling on the Board of Directors of the College to rescind a 1971 statement which stipulated that abortions should be performed only by physicians. On this, and the prospect of nurse-midwives performing abortions, see Lisa Summers, "The Genesis of the ACNM 1971 Statement on Abortion," *Journal of Nurse-Midwifery* 37 (1992): 168–74.

26. Mary Anne Freedman, David Jilson, Roberta Coffin, and Lloyd Novick, "Comparison of Complication Rates in First Trimester Abortions Performed by Physician Assistants and Physicians," *American Journal of Public Health* 76 (1986): 550–54.

27. On this point generally see Eliot Freidson, "Professional Dominance and the Ordering of Health Services," in his *Professional Dominance: The Social Structure of Medical Care* (New York: Atherton, 1970), pp. 127–66.

28. A strong boost to the efforts of nonphysicians to provide abortions came in a recent (1993) federal court decision in Montana which affirmed the legality of physician assistants performing abortions under the supervision of a physician. Donna Liberman and Anita Lalwani, "Physician-Only and Physician Assistant Statutes: A Case of Perceived but Unfounded Conflict," *Journal of the American Women's Medical Association* 49 (1994): 146–49.

29. National Abortion Federation, *Who Will Provide Abortions?*, p. 21.

30. The average pay for cardiovascular surgeons in private group practice was estimated in 1993 to be $574,769, while that of ob/gyns was $173,884 and family practitioners, $119,186. Erik Eckholm, "Health Plan is Toughest on Doctors Making Most," *New York Times*, November 7, 1993, pp. A1, A24.

31. David Grimes, "Clinicians Who Provide Abortions: The Thinning Ranks," *Obstetrics and Gynecology* 80 (1992): 719–23.

32. *Ibid.*, p. 722.

33. On the Abu Hayat case, see Lisa Belkin, "7 More Patients Accuse Doctor of Botching Their Abortions," *New York Times*, November 21, 1991, pp. B1, B12; and *ibid.*, "State Suspends Manhattan Doctor Accused of Botching Abortions," *New York Times*, November 26, 1991, pp. B1, B4.

34. UCSF Medical Students, "Letter to Life Dynamics," July 15, 1993. On abortion-related mobilization among medical students, see Jody Steinauer, *Abortion Action Guide: Medical Students for Choice* (Washington, D.C.: National Abortion Federation, 1993).

35. Carol S. Weisman, Constance A. Nathanson, Martha Ann Teitelbaum, Gary A. Chase, and Theodore King, in "Abortion Attitudes and Performance Among Male and Female Obstetrician-Gynecologists," *Family Planning Perspectives* 18 (1986): 67–72, report that "recently trained female obstetrician-gynecologists in active practice have more favorable attitudes toward abortion than do recently trained male ob/gyns, and the former are more likely to provide abortions" (p. 67). A similar finding of greater sympathy toward abortion among female physicians was reported in an American College of Obstetricians and Gynecologists poll of its members in 1985. ACOG, "Abortion Attitudes: Little Change in 14 Years," Washington, D.C., August 28, 1985.

Index

Abortionists, 32, 38, 45, 49; competent, 40–43, 66; illegal, 59, 99,
109–19; incompetent, 59, 62;
lay, 29, 31, 116–17; society, 78;
stigma associated with, 50–51,
53, 76, 152–53, 159

Accreditation Council of Gradu-
ate Medical Education
(ACGME), Residency Review
Committee for Obstetrics and
Gynecology of, 197

AFDC, 128, 166

AID (Agency for International
Development), 45–46

AIDS, 67

Ambulatory surgery, freestanding abortion clinics and, 42

American Association for Hospital Planning, 49

American Board of Obstetrics and
Gynecology, 197

American Civil Liberties Union,
166

American College of Obstetricians
and Gynecologists (ACOG), 4,
15–16, 24, 50, 157, 176; -NAF symposium, 196–97, 198, 201

American Law Institute (ALI), 39,
128

American Medical Association
(AMA), 35, 46, 47, 134; antiabor-

tion campaign of, 27–30; Committee on Criminal Abortion
of, 29; Council on Scientific
Affairs of, 4; founding of, 28;
House of Delegates of, 49

American Public Health Association (APHA), 49–50; *Comprehensive Guide for Abortion
Services*, 50

Anastomosis, end to end, 119

Anesthesia, 84, 94, 109, 115, 141; paracervical block, 135, 136

Antiabortion movement, 51–52,
109, 141, 202; harassment by,
and abortion practice, 161–73,
205; rise of militant, 6, 144; and
RU-486, 191; splits within, 187,
188; terrorist wing of, 2, 5, 162,
187, 188, 205, 207; and violence
and abortion provision, 187–89

Antibiotics, use of, after outpatient abortion, 18, 55, 117

Antistalking legislation, 188

Association for the Study of Abortion (ASA), 38–39; Hot Springs
conference of, 39–40, 41, 42, 44,
47, 76, 130, 135

Association of American Medical
Colleges, 49

Association of Reproductive
Health Professionals, 176

Baptists, Southern, 169–70
Barrett, James, 5, 187, 188
Barrington, Caleb, 68, 113–15, 143, 144, 156; and antiabortion harassment, 164–65; participation of, in abortion case, 176
Baulieu, Etienne, 190
Becker, Marshall, 48–49
Belous, Leon, 108
Bennett, Anna, 174–75
Bennett, David, 101, 143–45, 153–54, 159, 197–98; abortion by request offered by, 86–95; and National Abortion Federation, 174–75, 176
Berry, Reginald, 56
Birth control, 25, 42, 44, 68, 79; parallel between abortion and, 34–36; policies on agenda at Mount Sinai Hospital, 75; RU-486 for, 190; and Margaret Sanger, 9, 35, 67, 75. *See also* Contraceptive services
Birth defects: rubella and, 33; thalidomide and, 32
Bishop, Harris, 157, 166
Black, Victor, 55, 121–22, 158
Blackmail attempts by patients, 93, 95
Blackmun, Harry, 23
Bloom, Ethel, 54, 71–72
"Bottom Feeders" pamphlet, 207
Breast cancer, 290
Britton, John, 5, 187, 188
Buckley, Taylor, 58, 59, 62–63, 110–11
Burdick, C. Lalor, 44
Bureau of Alcohol, Tobacco and Firearms, 2
"Burnout," 173
Bush, George, 51, 187, 188, 189, 190
Butyric acid, 172

California, University of, at San Francisco Medical School, 157, 207

California Board of Medical Examiners, 33
Canadian Abortion Law (1969), 103, 105
Canadian Humanist Association, 97
Cannula, Karman, 45, 131, 141
Carleton College, 9, 22–23
Carter, Jimmy, 51
Casey, see *Planned Parenthood v. Casey*
Catholics, 11–12, 164, 166, 171, 178, 188. *See also* Roman Catholic church
Center for Reproductive and Sexual Health (Women's Services), 132–33, 136–38
Citizens for Abortion Reform, 129
Civil Liberties Union (Canada), 100
Clergy Consultation Service (CCS), 10, 92, 93, 95, 102, 203; Center for Reproductive and Sexual Health of, 132–33; domestic and international referrals by, 88–90, 113–15, 117; volunteers at, 136
Clinton, Bill, 1, 187, 189, 190, 194
Colposcopies, 201
Columbia Medical School, 137, 157
Columbia University, 3–4
Commitment to abortion work, sustaining, 173–78
Comstock laws, 34, 35
Confidentiality, issue of, 196
Constitution, U.S., 124
Contraceptive services, 181, 196, 206; at Preterm clinic, 147, 148. *See also* Birth control
Cost of abortion, 203. *See also* Payment for abortion
Costs, professional, of abortion work, 145–61
Counseling, abortion, 94, 133, 134–35, 147, 150, 201; effect of RU-

486 on, 192–93; provisions, mandated, 185
Criminalization of abortion, 28–32, 34, 47
Cushing's Syndrome, 190

D. & C., 11 and n, 14, 41, 54, 55, 140; combined method of vacuum suction and, 101; for illegal abortions, 58, 61, 76, 81, 91, 99, 131; following miscarriage, 33, 56; unwarranted, for retained tissue, 160; vs. vacuum suction method of abortion, 43, 76
Darney, Philip, 50–51
Darrow, Thomas, 64, 74, 169–71, 179
Davidson, Joe, 73–74
Deaths, from illegal abortions, 4, 29
Delay requirements, 184–85, 186
Diefenbaker, John, 104
Duluth (MN) Women's Health Center, 21, 26

Ehrlich, Ron, 129–30, 145, 155–56, 173, 178; and antiabortion harassment, 165–66
Eisenhower, Dwight, 44
Eisenstadt v. Baird, 35
England, abortions in, 37, 112, 113

FACE legislation (Freedom of Access to Clinic Entrance), 187, 189
Facilities, abortion, violent incidents at, 2, 5, 187–89. See also Freestanding abortion clinics
Family planning, 44–46, 52, 65–66, 79, 80, 101
FBI, 102, 187
FDA, 190
Fees, see Payment for abortion
Feminism, 39, 179. See also Women's movement

Fibroids, uterine, 41
Fieldstone, Daniel, 134–36, 141–42, 152, 154, 155, 157; and National Abortion Federation, 176; on need for program of reproductive health, 181–82; his pattern of providing illegal abortions, 74–78; on unintended pregnancies, 206
Finkbine, Sherri, 32, 33
Firebombings, 2, 5, 163, 188, 189
First District Court, 137
Fischer, Morris, 64, 126–27, 143, 144, 145–46, 181
Fox, Eugene, 59, 64–65, 69, 145, 152, 175; and antiabortion harassment, 166, 168; on obstetrics vs. abortion, 177–78
Freeman, Horace, 57, 64, 109, 122; and antiabortion harassment, 162, 163, 168
Freestanding abortion clinics, 24, 132–33, 141, 156, 158, 178; antiabortion harassment at, 5, 162; cost-driven reliance on, 195; enthusiasm about, 142, 146–47; increasing dependence on, 51, 134–35; marginality of abortion providers and success of, 160–61; as model of medical service delivery, 142, 144, 147; paracervical block used at, 135, 136; payment for abortions in, 203–4; reluctance of mainstream physicians about, 151–52; safety of abortions in, 138. See also Preterm clinic
Freestanding birth center, 178

Gag rule, 52
Gas gangrene, 60
Geiser, Lionel, 74
Generation, new, of abortion providers, 183, 206–8
German measles, see Rubella

Giardino, Renee, 60–61, 65–66

Glaucoma, 190

Goodman, Irving, 54–55, 59, 123, 158–59; his commitment to abortion provision, 82–86

Gordon, Ken, 57–58, 71, 145, 157, 173–74, 180

"Gray area" abortions, 124, 144, 185–86

Great Depression, 69

Greene, Rosalind, 61–62, 113, 124–25, 180

Grimes, David, 203, 204

Griswold v. Connecticut, 34–35

Gunn, David, 5, 187, 188, 189, 207

Guttmacher, Alan, 37, 38, 40, 42, 47; on abortions in outpatient facilities, 132; students of, 65, 75, 76

Hall, Robert, 47, 49

Harkin, Miriam, 61, 71, 115–17, 123, 146–47; and antiabortion harassment, 167; her dealings with therapeutic abortion committees, 120–21; tradeoff made by, 177

Harmon, Judith, 136–38, 151–52, 167

Harris, Zachary, 163, 168

Harvard Medical School, 157

Harvey, Hale, 132, 137

Hayat, Abu, 204–5

Health care reform, 2, 183, 194–96

Hemolysis, 59

HMO (health maintenance organization), 166

Hodgson, Jane, 96, 134, 160, 201; arrest and trial of, 14–15; conviction and appeal of, 17–18; Defense Fund for, 14; early medical practice of, 9–11, 12; illegal abortion performed by, 8, 14, 17; involvement of, in legalizing abortion, 11–26; and Preterm clinic, 18–19; *Roe v.*

Wade's impact on conviction of, 19; semiretirement of, 25–26

Hodgson v. Minnesota, 21

Hoechst AG, 190

Hospital(s): -based abortion activity in pre-*Roe* era, 119–27; immense demands placed on, by illegal abortion, 56–61; percentage of all abortions taking place in, 161; presence of police in, 61–62

Humanism, 179

Humanist Fellowship of Montreal, 97–98

Hyde Amendment, 194–95

Hyperplasia, 74

Hypnosis, 94

Hysterectomy, 3, 71

Illegal abortionists, *see* Abortionists

IUDs (intrauterine devices), 66, 67–68, 79–81, 117

Jacobs, George, 114, 127–28, 157

Japan, abortions in, 37, 112, 113, 114, 121

Johns Hopkins University, 40

Joint Commission on Accreditation of Hospitals, 49

Karman, Harvey, 45, 131, 141

Kaufman, Marty, 143–44, 175–76

Kenslake, Dorothea, 44, 131

Kinsey Report, 29

Lader, Lawrence, 37, 137

Lalor Foundation, 44, 131, 135

Lamm, Richard, 128

Legal climate, 184–86

Legalization, *see Roe v. Wade*

Legal uncertainty, 30–37

Leunbach paste, 41, 59

Lever, Ed, 62, 63, 113, 125, 128, 154–55; and antiabortion harassment, 166, 167

Levin, Harry, 147, 148
Lewit, Sarah, 138
Litmus tests, abortion, 51–52
Lowney, Shannon, 5, 188
Lucas, Roy, 15
Luker, Kristin, 36

McCrae v. Harris, 21
McKelvey, John, 15
McPherson, Peters, 57
Madsen v. Women's Health Ser-vices, 188
Maginnis, Pat, 78
Malpractice, 2, 21, 190; law firms specializing in abortion, 189
Managed care, 195, 196
Marginalization, of abortion practice from mainstream medicine, 6, 144, 160–61, 173, 195, 204
"Maternity homes," 10
Mayo Clinic, 9, 16
Meadows, Tania, 45, 53–54, 63–64, 111–12
Medicaid, 20, 26, 48, 122; recipients, federal funding of abortions for, 51, 204
Medical abortion, 189–94
Medical Committee for Human Rights, 128, 136
Medical equivocation, *Roe* decision and, 46–52
Medical mobilization for legal abortion, 38–46
"Medical Students for Choice," 207
Meningiomas, 190
"Menstrual extraction kits," 44–45
Mental health considerations, abortion and, 32, 36, 37, 121–22
Messinger, Barry, 130–32, 147, 151
Methotrexate, 193–94
Mexico, abortions in, 37, 111–12, 113, 117
Midwest Health Clinic for Women, 20

Midwives, *see* Nurse midwives
Minnesota, University of, 9, 15, 16, 20, 22
Minnesota Medicine, 12
Minnesota Obstetrical/Gynecological Society, 8, 10, 16, 22
Miscarriage, 33, 34, 56, 57, 87, 145
Misoprostol, 193–94
Montreal, University of, 96
Morgentaler, Henry, 21, 86, 197–98, 202; his activism on behalf of abortion reform in Canada, 95–103, 105–7; jailing of, 104–5; raids on clinics of, 102, 105; trials of, 102, 103–4
Morgentaler, Josef, 96
Morgentaler Amendment, 104, 105
Mount Sinai Hospital (Baltimore), 37
Mount Sinai Hospital (NYC), 75–76, 77
Murders, at abortion facilities, 5, 187, 188, 189, 207

NARAL, 137
Nathanson, Constance, 48–49
National Abortion Federation (NAF), 4, 96, 174–75, 176, 207; -ACOG symposium, 196–97, 198, 201; annual meetings of, 1–3, 209
National Board of Medical Examiners, 49
National Conference of Catholic Bishops, 188
National Right to Life Committee, 188
Network, national, of medical abortion activists, 130
New York Academy of Medicine, 36
Nichols, Leanne, 5, 188
Novak, Franc, 43–44
Nurse midwives, 29, 198, 200
Nurse practitioners, 198, 200

Obstetrics and gynecology (ob/
    gyn) program: lack of abortion
    training in, 3–4, 48, 197, 199;
    mandated training in abortion
    techniques in, 208
Ogden, Stan, 166–67
Oliver, Stan, 57
Omnibus Crime Bill of 1994, 188
Operation Rescue, 6, 162, 189

Pacific Coast Ob/Gyn Society, 155
Pain management, 94, 174
Paracervical block, 135, 136
Pathfinder Fund, 150
Payment for abortion, 85, 93–94,
    100, 124–25, 140; ambivalence
    about, 81–82; confronting com-
    plex question of, 202–4
Peritonitis, 55
Phillips, Bob, 138–39, 152–53, 180,
    181
Physician assistants (PAs), 198,
    199–200
Picketing, by antiabortionists,
    162–64, 165, 166, 167, 171, 173
Pill, abortion, *see* RU-486
Planned Parenthood, 34, 44, 132,
    139–40; abortion training pro-
    grams at, 198, 200; antiabor-
    tion harassment at, 164, 165;
    conference of, 39–40, 130; of
    Minnesota, 20; on need for
    changes in abortion policy, 39
Planned Parenthood v. Casey, 1,
    184, 185, 186
Pneumonia, pneumocystic
    occurring, 67
Pool of abortion providers,
    expanding, 198–200
Population control, 44, 46
Population Council, 147, 191
Potassium permanganate tablets,
    34, 57
Pregnancy test, early, 9
Pregnant woman, as ultimate
    decisionmaker, 180

Presbyterian church, 170
Preterm clinic (Washington,
    D.C.), 18–19, 39, 134, 137; Ethan
    Stevenson's experiences at,
    147–51, 175. *See also* Freestand-
    ing abortion clinics
Procedures, increasing repertoire
    of clinic medical, 201
"Pro-choice," range of feelings
    covered by phrase, 178–80
Project Hope, 11
Prostaglandin, 189, 193
Protestant clergy, 28
Provider shortage, responses of
    medical community to, 196–
    204
Public Health Service, U.S., 66
Puerto Rico, abortions in, 37, 111,
    112, 113

Quattlebaum, Francis, 11
Quebec Court of Appeal, 103–4

Radical health movements, 46
Reagan, Ronald, 45, 51, 187, 188
Referrals, abortion, 109–17, 125–26,
    133, 140, 158–59
Regulation of abortion services,
    184–86
Relaxation techniques, 94
Reno, Janet, 187
Reproductive freedom, 25, 48, 168,
    181
Reproductive health, need for pro-
    gram of, 181–82
Roe v. Wade, 6, 7, 14, 71; and Harry
    Blackmun, 23; challenge to, 4;
    impact of, 8–9, 146; impact of,
    on conviction of Jane Hodg-
    son, 19; Roy Lucas's con-
    tribution to, 15; medical
    equivocation and, 46–52;
    Supreme Court's decision in, 1,
    143–45, 184
Roman Catholic church, 28, 65,
    129. *See also* Catholics

Roots, Margaret, 67–68
Ross, Simon, 65, 66–68, 84, 179, 202; his decision to provide illegal abortions, 78–82
Rotary Club, 40, 92
Rothstein, Sheldon, 72–73, 112, 117–19, 122
Roussel-Uclaf, 190
Routinization of abortion work, 151
Rubella, 13, 15, 72, 84, 121, 127; and birth defects, 33
RU-486 (mifepristone), 183, 189–93, 194, 200, 208

St. Paul-Ramsey Hospital (MN), 14, 20, 22
Saline injection method of abortion, 80, 81, 130
"San Francisco Nine," 32, 33, 38
Sanger, Margaret, 9, 35, 36, 67, 75
Septicemia, 58, 60
Septic shock, 57–58, 83
Smith, Peter, 71
Social class, accessibility of abortion and, 36, 48–49
Spencer, Robert, 40–43, 45, 50–51, 59, 117–18
Spontaneous abortion, 33, 56, 77, 87
Sterilization, 37, 75, 147
Stevenson, Ethan, 147, 201; experiences of, at Preterm clinic, 147–51, 175
Stone, Hannah, 36
Strangulated hernia, 58
Sulfa drugs, 41
Supreme Court, Minnesota, 14, 17–18
Supreme Court, U.S., 14, 21, 23, 124, 176, 189; and Comstock laws, 34; on federal funding of abortions for Medicaid recipients, 51; and *Madsen v. Women's Health Services*, 188; and *Planned Parenthood v. Casey*, 1, 184; and *Roe v. Wade*, 1, 143–45, 184; and *Webster v. Reproductive Health Services*, 4
Supreme Court of Canada, 104, 105
Sweden, abortions in, 32, 112
Swensen, Charles, 112, 121, 129, 138, 139–40, 181; costs of abortion work to, 153, 155
Swinton, Bill, 163, 168–69

Taussig, Frederick, 29
Teenagers, parental notification and consent requirements for, 184, 186
Temple, Paul, 157, 158, 179
Terrorism, antiabortion, 2, 5, 162, 187, 188, 205, 207
Thalidomide, 32
Therapeutic abortion committees, 10, 36–37, 63–64, 70; appointment of abortion-sympathetic doctors to, 123; hospital-based abortions approved by, 119–27, 129; at Mount Sinai Hospital, 75
Third World, 11, 44, 45
Thomas, Louise, 60, 65, 177
Tietze, Christopher, 15, 138
Timanus, L. Cottrell, 40, 41, 42, 45, 50–51
Truman, Harry, 44

Unitarian Church, 87, 88, 89
Uterus: injecting saline solution into, 80, 81, 130; irritation of, and pregnancy rate, 79; perforation of, 43, 58, 59, 205

Vacuum suction method of abortion, 76, 91, 100–101, 130–32, 135–36, 141; introduction of, 43–45
Vasectomies, 79, 81
Vermont, University of, 198
Vermont Women's Health Center, 198

Vietnam War, 88, 92
Violence, and abortion provision,
    187–89, 210

Waiting periods, 184–85, 186
Washington Hospital Center, 137
Watson, Alice, 171, 172
Watson, Oswald, 162–63, 171–72
*Webster v. Reproductive Health Ser-
    vices,* 4
Wellstone, Howard, 69, 125–26

Widmeyer, Nancy, 13–14
Wilkins, Alice, 56, 71
Williams, Buck, 184
Women's health movement, 46,
    133–34, 141
Women's movement, 25, 52
Women's Services, *see* Center for
    Reproductive and Sexual
    Health
World War I, 35, 118
World War II, 36, 42, 59, 74